Achieving Cultural Competency

Commissioning Editor: Mary Banks
Development Editor: Laura Quigley
Editorial Assistant: Lewis O'Sullivan

Achieving Cultural Competency

A case-based approach to training health professionals

EDITORS-IN-CHIEF
Lisa Hark, PhD, RD
Consultant, Department of Medicine
Jefferson Medical College
Thomas Jefferson University
Philadelphia, PA, USA

Horace DeLisser, MD
Associate Professor of Medicine in Pulmonary, Allergy and Critical Care
Assistant Dean, Cultural Competency and Spirituality
University of Pennsylvania School of Medicine
Philadelphia, PA, USA

SENIOR EDITOR
Gail Morrison, MD
Vice Dean of Education
Professor of Medicine
University of Pennsylvania School of Medicine
Philadelphia, PA, USA

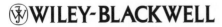

WILEY-BLACKWELL
A John Wiley & Sons, Ltd., Publication

This edition first published 2009, © 2009 by Blackwell Publishing Ltd

Blackwell Publishing was acquired by John Wiley & Sons in February 2007. Blackwell's publishing program has been merged with Wiley's global Scientific, Technical and Medical business to form Wiley-Blackwell.

Registered office: John Wiley & Sons Ltd, The Atrium, Southern Gate, Chichester, West Sussex, PO19 8SQ, UK

Editorial offices: 9600 Garsington Road, Oxford, OX4 2DQ, UK
       The Atrium, Southern Gate, Chichester, West Sussex, PO19 8SQ, UK
       111 River Street, Hoboken, NJ 07030-5774, USA

For details of our global editorial offices, for customer services and for information about how to apply for permission to reuse the copyright material in this book please see our website at www.wiley.com/wiley-blackwell

The right of the author to be identified as the author of this work has been asserted in accordance with the Copyright, Designs and Patents Act 1988.

Wiley also publishes its books in a variety of electronic formats. Some content that appears in print may not be available in electronic books.

Designations used by companies to distinguish their products are often claimed as trademarks. All brand names and product names used in this book are trade names, service marks, trademarks or registered trademarks of their respective owners. The publisher is not associated with any product or vendor mentioned in this book. This publication is designed to provide accurate and authoritative information in regard to the subject matter covered. It is sold on the understanding that the publisher is not engaged in rendering professional services. If professional advice or other expert assistance is required, the services of a competent professional should be sought.

The contents of this work are intended to further general scientific research, understanding, and discussion only and are not intended and should not be relied upon as recommending or promoting a specific method, diagnosis, or treatment by physicians for any particular patient. The publisher and the author make no representations or warranties with respect to the accuracy or completeness of the contents of this work and specifically disclaim all warranties, including without limitation any implied warranties of fitness for a particular purpose. In view of ongoing research, equipment modifications, changes in governmental regulations, and the constant flow of information relating to the use of medicines, equipment, and devices, the reader is urged to review and evaluate the information provided in the package insert or instructions for each medicine, equipment, or device for, among other things, any changes in the instructions or indication of usage and for added warnings and precautions. Readers should consult with a specialist where appropriate. The fact that an organization or Website is referred to in this work as a citation and/or a potential source of further information does not mean that the author or the publisher endorses the information the organization or Website may provide or recommendations it may make. Further, readers should be aware that Internet Websites listed in this work may have changed or disappeared between when this work was written and when it is read. No warranty may be created or extended by any promotional statements for this work. Neither the publisher nor the author shall be liable for any damages arising herefrom.

Library of Congress Cataloging-in-Publication Data

Achieving cultural competency : a case-based approach to training health professionals / editors-in-chief, Lisa Hark, Horace DeLisser ; senior editor, Gail Morrison.
   p. ; cm.
Includes bibliographical references.
ISBN 978-1-4051-8072-6
1. Transcultural medical care–Case studies.   2. Physician and patient–Case studies.
3. Medical personnel–Training of–Case studies.   I. Hark, Lisa. II. DeLisser, Horace.
III. Morrison, Gail.
   [DNLM: 1. Cultural Competency–Case Reports.   2. Ethics, Clinical–Case Reports.
3. Physician-Patient Relations–Case Reports.   4. Prejudice–Case Reports. W 21 A178 2009]
RA418.5.T73A24 2009
610.69'6–dc22

                            2008039954

A catalogue record for this book is available from the British Library.

Set in 9.25/12 pt Meridien by Aptara® Inc., New Delhi, India
Printed and bound in Singapore by Fabulous Printers Pte Ltd

1   2009

Contents

Contributors

Associate Editors

Olivia Carter-Pokras, PhD
Associate Professor
Department of Epidemiology and Biostatistics
University of Maryland School of Public Health
College Park, MD, USA

Darwin Deen, MD, MS
Medical Professor
Department of Community Health and Social Medicine
Sophie Davis College of Biomedical Education
City College of New York, NY, USA

Desiree Lie, MD, MSEd
Clinical Professor of Family Medicine
Department of Family Medicine
University of California at Irvine, Orange, CA, USA

Ana Núñez, MD
Director of Women's Health Education Program
Associate Professor of Medicine
Drexel University College of Medicine, Philadelphia, PA, USA

Debbie Salas-Lopez, MD, MPH, FACP
Associate Professor of Medicine
Division of General Internal Medicine
Vice Chair of Medicine
Lehigh Valley Hospital and Health Network, Allentown, PA, USA

Helen Abramova, MD, Postdoctoral Research Fellow, Division of Pulmonary, Allergy, and Critical Care Medicine, University of Pennsylvania School of Medicine, Philadelphia, PA, USA

Thomas A. Arcury, PhD, Professor and Research Director, Department of Family and Community Medicine Wake Forest University School of Medicine, Winston-Salem, NC, USA

Elena N. Atochina-Vasserman, MD, PhD, Senior Research Investigator, Division of Pulmonary, Allergy, and Critical Care Medicine University of Pennsylvania School of Medicine, Philadelphia, PA, USA

Lisa Bellini, MD, Professor of Pulmonary, Allergy, and Critical Care Medicine, University of Pennsylvania School of Medicine, Philadelphia, PA, USA

Clarence H. Braddock III, MD, MPH, Associate Dean for Medical Education Stanford University School of Medicine, Stanford, CA, USA

Fran Burke, MS, RD, Senior Clinical Dietitian, Department of Cardiovascular Medicine University of Pennsylvania School of Medicine, Philadelphia, PA, USA

Olivia Carter-Pokras, PhD, Associate Professor, Department of Epidemiology and Biostatistics University of Maryland School of Public Health, College Park, MD, USA

Alexander J. Chou, MD, Instructor, Department of Pediatrics Memorial Sloan-Kettering Cancer Center, New York, NY, USA

April Coleman, Managing Editor University of Pennsylvania School of Medicine, Philadelphia, PA, USA

Ronald G. Collman, MD, Professor of Pulmonary, Allergy, and Critical Care Medicine; Co-director, Penn Center for AIDS Research, University of Pennsylvania School of Medicine, Philadelphia, PA, USA

Nereida Correa, MD, MPH, Associate Clinical Professor of OB/GYN and Women's Health, Albert Einstein College of Medicine, Bronx, NY, USA

Sonia Crandall, PhD, MS, Professor of Family and Community Medicine Wake Forest University School of Medicine, Winston-Salem, NC, USA

Hetty Cunningham, MD, Assistant Clinical Professor of Pediatrics Columbia University College of Physicians and Surgeons, New York, NY, USA

Horace DeLisser, MD, Associate Professor of Pulmonary, Allergy, and Spiritual Care Medicine; Assistant Dean, Cultural Competency University of Pennsylvania School of Medicine, Philadelphia, PA, USA

Sharon Drozdowsky, MES, Industrial Hygienist, Consultation, Education and Outreach Services, Division of Occupational Safety and Health Washington State Department of Labor and Industries, Tumwater, WA, USA

Eric J. Gertner, MD, MPH, Associate Professor of Clinical Medicine Lehigh Valley Hospital and Health Network, Allentown, PA, USA

Indira Gurubhagavatula, MD, Assistant Professor of Sleep, Pulmonary, Allergy, and Critical Care, Medicine University of Pennsylvania School of Medicine, Veteran Affairs Medical Center of Philadelphia, PA, USA

Roy Hamilton, MD, MS, Assistant Professor of Neurology University of Pennsylvania School of Medicine, Philadelphia, PA, USA

Lisa Hark, PhD, RD, Consultant, Department of Medicine, Jefferson Medical College, Thomas Jefferson University, Philadelphia, PA, USA

Scott Kasner, MD, Associate Professor of Neurology; Director Comprehensive Stroke Center University of Pennsylvania School of Medicine, Philadelphia, PA, USA

Nadine T. Katz, MD, Associate Dean for Students; Associate Professor and Director of Medical Education, Department of Obstetrics and Gynecology and Women's Health Albert Einstein College of Medicine, Bronx, New York, NY, USA

Amal Mohamed Osman Khidir, MD, FAAP, Assistant Professor of Pediatrics; Director, Pediatric Clerkship Weill Cornell Medical College in Qatar, Doha, Qatar

Lyuba Konopasek, MD, Associate Professor of Pediatrics (Education); Course Director, Medicine, Patients, and Society; Director, Pediatric Undergraduate Education Weill Cornell Medical College, New York, NY, USA

Elizabeth Lee-Rey, MD, MPH, Assistant Professor of Family and Social Medicine; Co-Director, Hispanic Center of Excellence Albert Einstein College of Medicine, Bronx, New York, NY, USA

Ryan Leonard, Research Assistant and Item Writer University of Pennsylvania School of Medicine, Philadelphia, PA, USA

Desiree Lie, MD, MSEd, Clinical Professor of Family Medicine, Department of Family Medicine University of California at Irvine, Orange, CA, USA

Edgar Maldonado, MD, Assistant Clinical Professor of Medicine; Medical Director, Centro de Salud Latino Americano and Diabetes Institute Lehigh Valley Hospital and Health Network, Allentown, PA, USA

Mitchell L. Margolis, MD, Director of Clinical Pulmonary Medicine Veterans Affairs Medical Center of Philadelphia, Philadelphia, PA, USA

Gail S. Marion, PA, PhD, Professor of Family and Community Medicine Wake Forest University Baptist Medical Center, Winston-Salem, NC, USA

Rica Mauricio, Former Health Education and Adult Literacy Program Coordinator and Researcher, Columbia University College of Physicians and Surgeons, New York, NY, USA

Steven R. Messé, MD, Assistant Professor of Neurology, University of Pennsylvania School of Medicine, Philadelphia, PA, USA

Dodi Meyer, MD, Associate Clinical Professor of Pediatrics Columbia University College of Physicians and Surgeons, New York, NY, USA

Ana Núñez, MD, Director of Women's Health Education Program; Associate Professor of Medicine Drexel University College of Medicine, Philadelphia, PA, USA

Sashank Prasad, MD, Instructor, University of Pennsylvania School of Medicine, Philadelphia, PA, USA

Noel B. Rosales, MD, Director, Cultural Effectiveness Initiative; Assistant Professor of Pediatrics Children's Hospital of Philadelphia, Philadelphia, PA, USA

Lisa Rucker, MD, Associate Professor of Clinical Medicine Albert Einstein College of Medicine, Bronx, NY, USA

J. Eric Russell, MD, Associate Professor of Medicine Pediatrics University of Pennsylvania School of Medicine, Philadelphia, PA, USA

Debbie Salas-Lopez, MD, MPH, FACP, Associate Professor of Medicine, Division of General Internal Medicine, Vice Chair of Medicine, Lehigh Valley Hospital and Health Network, Allentown, PA, USA

John Paul Sánchez, MD, MPH, Emergency Medicine Resident Jacobi Medical Center, Albert Einstein College of Medicine, Bronx, NY, USA

Nelson Felix Sánchez, MD, Instructor, Department of Internal Medicine, Memorial Sloan-Kettering Cancer Center, New York, NY, USA

Alexandra Schieber, Medical Student, New York University School of Medicine, New York, NY, USA

Nicholas E. S. Sibinga, MD, Associate Professor of Medicine (Cardiology) Albert Einstein College of Medicine, New York, NY, USA

Charles Vega, MD, FAAFP, Associate Clinical Professor of Family Medicine; Director, Program in Medical Education for the Latino Community University of California at Irvine, Irving, CA, USA

Susan E. Wiegers, MD, Professor of Cardiovascular Medicine University of Pennsylvania School of Medicine, Philadelphia, PA, USA

Achieving Cultural Competency: A Case-Based Approach to Training Health Professionals

Directions for Continuing Medical Education Credits

Duration: Maximum of 25 hours, each case should take 1 hour
Credit: Up to 25 *AMA PRA Category 1 Credits*™, each case is awarded 1 *AMA PRA Category 1 Credit*™

Original Release Date: June 1, 2009
Last Review Date: January 5, 2009
Expiration: May 31, 2012

There is no commercial support for this activity.

Program Overview: *Achieving Cultural Competency: A Case-Based Approach to Training Health Professionals* will provide the necessary tools to meet the ever growing need that health professionals in training and practice have to become culturally competent. A total of 25 self-study clinical cases will be presented on a variety of medical topics, including cardiovascular, endocrine, pulmonary, neurology, oncology, hematology, immunology, OB-GYN, and pediatric disorders. Learners will not only gain knowledge, but will have direct insight into real life, actual scenarios that have occurred in clinical settings. Cultural factors covered within the cases include cultural diversity plus gender, language, folk beliefs, socioeconomic status, health literacy, religion, and sexual orientation.

Intended Audience: This activity has been designed for physicians in training (interns, residents and fellows), practicing physicians and is also applicable to all medical disciplines and specialties and medical students.

Overall Educational Objectives
Upon completion of this activity, participants should be better able to:
1 Describe the language, culture, and behaviors of diverse individuals and their families.
2 Examine self-awareness and knowledge of the cultural factors that may affect interactions between patients and health care providers.
3 Employ skills to provide culturally effective and appropriate healthcare.

Accreditation: The University of Pennsylvania School of Medicine is accredited by the Accreditation Council for Continuing Medical Education (ACCME) to provide continuing medical education for physicians.

Directions for Continuing Medical Education Credits

Designation of Credit: The University of Pennsylvania School of Medicine designates this educational activity for a maximum of

25 *AMA PRA Category 1 Credits*^{TM}. Each case in this activity is designated for a maximum of 1 *AMA PRA Category 1 Credit*^{TM}. Physicians should only claim credit commensurate with the extent of their participation in the activity.

Disclosures: It is policy at the University of Pennsylvania School of Medicine for individuals who are in a position to control the content of an educational activity to disclose to the learners all relevant financial relationships that they have with any commercial interest that provides products or services that may be relevant to the content of this continuing medical education activity.

The staff in the Office of CME at the University of Pennsylvania School of Medicine and the peer reviewer, Zalman Agus, MD, have reported **no relevant** financial relationships with any commercial interests related to the content of this educational activity.

The faculty/editors listed below have disclosed that they have **no relevant** financial relationships with any commercial interests related to the content of this educational activity.

Helen Abramova, MD
Thomas A. Arcury, PhD
Elena Atochina-Vasserman, MD, PhD
Lisa Bellini, MD
Clarence H. Braddock III, MD, MPH
Frances Burke, MS, RD
Olivia Carter-Pokras, PhD
Alexander Chou, MD
April Coleman
Ronald G. Collman, MD
Nereida Correa, MD, MPH
Sonia Crandall, PhD, MS
Hetty Cunningham, MD
Darwin Deen, MD, MS
Horace DeLisser, MD
Sharon Drozdowsky, MES
Eric J. Gertner, MD, MPH
Indira Gurubhagavatula, MD
Roy Hamilton, MD, MS
Lisa Hark, PhD, RD
Scott Kasner, MD
Nadine T. Katz, MD
Amal Mohamed Osman Khidir, MD, FAAP

Lyuba Konopasek, MD
Elizabeth Lee-Rey, MD, MPH
Ryan Leonard
Desiree Lie, MD, MSEd
Edgar Maldonado, MD
Mitchell Margolis, MD
Gail Marion, PA-C, PhD
Rica Mauricio
Steven R. Messé, MD
Dodi Meyer, MD
Gail Morrison, MD
Ana Nunez, MD
Sashank Prasad, MD
Noel B. Rosales, MD
Lisa Rucker, MD
J. Eric Russell, MD
Debbie Salas-Lopez, MD, MPH, FACP
John Paul Sánchez, MD, MPH
Nelson Felix Sánchez, MD
Alexandra Schieber
Nicholas E. S. Sibinga, MD
Charles Vega, MD, FAAFP
Susan E. Wiegers, MD

Investigational and/or Off-Label Use of Commercial Products and Devices: The University of Pennsylvania School of Medicine requires all faculty to disclose any planned discussion of an investigational and/or off-label use of a pharmaceutical product or device within their presentation. Participants should note that the use of products outside FDA-approved labeling should be considered experimental and are advised to consult current prescribing information for approved indications.

The faculty members listed above have reported that there will be no discussion of investigational and/or off-label use of commercial products within the activity.

Completion Instructions

- To receive CME credit for each case that you complete from this book, please visit the University of Pennsylvania Office of Continuing Medical Education website at: http://www.med.upenn.edu/cme/culture/
- Once on the site, you will be presented with the option to choose from two topics. The topic for this book is called "Achieving Cultural Competency Book Cases (Wiley-Blackwell 2009)". After choosing this topic, you will be presented **with a complete list of cases from this book.**
  Select the case(s) for which you would like to receive CME credit.
- In order to access any of these cases, you must have an account on the CME Website (complementary).
- If you *do not* have an account, sign-up (click on **member sign-up** at the top of the page).
- If you have an account, log into the site with your e-mail address and password (click on **log-in** at the top of the page).
- Next, register for a particular activity (case) by using the link in the "Course Materials" box on the right. When prompted for an access code, enter: **culturebook** (Note: the access code is case-sensitive).
- Click on the "Get CME" link in the "Course Materials" box.
- You now need to complete the Post-Test.
- After successfully completing the Post-Test, with a **score of 75% or higher**, you will be directed to the Evaluation.
- After completing the Evaluation, you will be able to view, print, or save a CME certificate verifying your credit for this activity.

Computer Requirements
Windows: Latest release of <u>Safari</u>, <u>Internet Explorer 6/7</u> or <u>Mozilla/Firefox</u>.
Macintosh: Latest release of <u>Safari</u> or <u>Mozilla/Firefox</u>.
Plugins: <u>Real Player</u>

Contact Information: For CME-related questions, please contact the University of Pennsylvania School of Medicine, Office of Continuing Medical Education, at penncme@mail.med.upenn.edu or at 215-898-9750.

Preface

We are extremely proud of the first edition of *Achieving Cultural Competency: A Case-Based Approach to Training Health Professionals*. We hope this book will provide the necessary tools to meet the ever-growing need that health professionals in training and practice have to become culturally competent. Twenty-five self-study cases are presented on a variety of medical topics in the areas of cardiovascular disease, pulmonary medicine, metabolic and endocrine diseases, obstetrics and gynecology, neurology, oncology, hematology, and pediatric disorders. Issues covered within the cases include cultural diversity plus gender, language, folk beliefs, socioeconomic status, religion, and sexual orientation. Learners will gain knowledge, and learn skills related to health disparities, community strategies, bias and stereotyping, communication skills, use of interpreters, and self-reflection as recommended by the AAMC's *Tools to Assess Cultural Competency Training*. Many health professionals have collaborated to write these cases that provide direct insights into real-life, actual scenarios that have occurred in clinical settings.

Culture is difficult to define and can easily be taken for granted. The pressures of modern medical practice are such that, as physicians treat their patients, they may tend to focus only on the medical issues, while neglecting the cultural heritage, beliefs, and values of their patients. Unfortunately, failure to consider and address these issues in the doctor–patient relationship may result in poor outcomes for individual patients, which may contribute to national health-related disparities for the entire society. We are pleased to be able to contribute this content and feel confident that, as physicians become more culturally competent, they will be able to provide better, more effective care to their patients. There is nothing more reassuring to patients than knowing that their health care provider respects and understands who they are as people, including the cultural factors that define them.

For this reason, the University of Pennsylvania School of Medicine, Office of Continuing Medical Education (CME) has recognized the importance of this material for physicians. The University of Pennsylvania School of Medicine is accredited by the Accreditation Council for Continuing Medical Education (ACCME) to provide continuing medical education for physicians.

The University of Pennsylvania School of Medicine designates each case of this educational activity for a maximum of 1 *AMA PRA Category 1 Credit*™. Physicians should only claim credit commensurate with the extent of their participation in the activity. Information about CME credits for this book can be found on pages xii and 219 and at the following Web site: http://www.med.upenn.edu/cme.

For more information about the University of Pennsylvania School of Medicine's Cultural Competency Medical Education Program, visit http://www.med.upenn.edu/culture.

Horace DeLisser, MD, Lisa Hark, PhD, RD and Gail Morrison, MD

Foreword

Clarence H. Braddock III, MD, MPH, FACP

In the early 1980s, there was increasing recognition of the powerful challenge that our health care system was facing in providing high-quality care to increasingly diverse populations. As a result, the term "cultural competence" entered the language of health professions education in the late 1980s. Based on the work of Cross and others, many authors began to articulate frameworks for defining cultural competence (1). Yet cultural competence was slow to emerge as an important fixture in health professions education.

A large part of this slow progress was the ongoing debate on defining cultural competence. Is cultural competence the knowledge of the unique traditions, health beliefs, and health of a defined population? Is it a set of communication skills to better understand the unique health needs and beliefs of any patient? Is it more of an attitude—a stance—in which the physician shows the humility and curiosity to explore the patient's background and allow what is learned to inform diagnosis and treatment? In reality, cultural competence is all these things. This recognition has stymied many educators seeking to develop curricula to address the challenge.

In 2000, the Liaison Committee for Medical Education, the organization that sets and applies accreditation standards for U.S. Medical Schools, added a standard for teaching about the role of culture in clinical practice:

> "The faculty and students must demonstrate an understanding of the manner in which people of diverse cultures and belief systems perceive health and illness and respond to various symptoms, diseases, and treatments. Medical students should learn to recognize and appropriately address gender and cultural biases in health care delivery, while considering first the health of the patient" (2).

In 2003, the Institute of Medicine (IOM) published its landmark report, *Unequal Treatment*. This publication cataloged the growing body of evidence of the vast extent of disparities in health care in the United States. The IOM recommended that health care profession education include specific training in cultural competence. These two strong statements drew attention to a previously overlooked area of education and training, and many educators began to scramble to find ways to teach cultural competence (3).

The cause of cultural competence education took a major step forward with the publication by the Association of American Medical College's *Tools for Assessing Cultural Competence Training (TACCT)* in 2005. Developed by a national expert panel of educators in this area, TACCT provides a framework of broad domains of cultural competence and 42 specific learning objectives for use in constructing a robust cultural competence curriculum (4).

Currently, the majority of health professions schools, postgraduate training programs, and health care systems are working to meet the goal of preparing a workforce who can deliver high-quality and culturally and linguistically appropriate care to all. The remaining challenge in cultural competence—and it is not a small one—is developing meaningful and effective strategies to teach cultural competence. There are a few Web-based resources, most notably the National Consortium for Multicultural Education for the Health Professions the University of Pennsylvania School of Medicine and the University of Alabama at Birmingham Web sites, but precious few textbooks or guides to teaching and learning in this area, until now (5–7). Hark and DeLisser's *Achieving Cultural Competency: A Case-Based Approach for Training Health Professionals* is a fabulous addition to the growing list of resources for teaching. The authors have assembled a rich resource, with contributions from many of the top educators in cultural competence in the United States.

This book fills an important niche, providing a rich and diverse set of cases for teaching and learning. By mapping the learning objectives of the cases to the TACCT, the authors and their contributors have added incredible value. The authors have masterfully molded their years of combined experience into a usable guide to case-based education in cultural competence. Now educators seeking to add curriculum on a particular TACCT domain or set of learning objectives can select high-quality materials for the kind of teaching that embraces principles of adult learning: experiential and case-based teaching (See pp. xxix and Appendix 3).

Achieving Cultural Competency: A Case-Based Approach for Training Health Professionals will undoubtedly become a fixture in the libraries of faculty in health professions schools who are charged to develop, expand, or augment their curriculum in cultural competence. I'm certain that the originators of the cultural competence movement would be gratified to see the kind of high-quality attention this topic is now receiving in health professions education.

Clarence H. Braddock III, MD, MPH, FACP
Associate Professor of Medicine
Associate Dean for Medical Education
Stanford University School of Medicine
Director, National Consortium for Multicultural Education for Health Professionals.

References

1. Cross T.L., Bazron B.J., Isaacs M.R., et al. *Towards a culturally competent system of care: A monograph on effective services for minority children who are severely emotionally disturbed.* Georgetown University Center for Child Health and Mental Health Policy, CASSP Technical Assistance Center, Washington DC, 1989.
2. Liaison Committee for Medical Education. *Functions and Structure of a Medical School: Standards for Accreditation of Medical Education Programs Leading to the M.D. Degree,* 2007.
3. Smedley B.D., Stith A.Y., Nelson A.R. *Unequal Treatment: Confronting Racial and Ethnic Disparities in Health Care.* Institute of Medicine (U.S.): Committee on Understanding and Eliminating Racial and Ethnic Disparities in Health Care. The National Academies Press, 2003.
4. Association of American Medical Colleges. Cultural Competence Education for Medical Students. 2005. Available at: http://www.aamc.org/meded/tacct/start.htm.
5. National Consortium for Multicultural Education for Health Professionals. Available at: http://culturalmeded.stanford.edu.
6. University of Pennsylvania School of Medicine's Cultural Competency Medical Education Program and Resources. Available at: http://www.med.upenn.edu/culture.
7. Cultural Competence Online for Medical Practice (CCOMP). A Clinician's Guide to Reduce Cardiovascular Disparities, especially hypertension, University of Alabama at Birmingham. Available at http://www.c-comp.org.

Acknowledgments

We gratefully acknowledge the National Heart, Lung, and Blood Institute at the NIH for providing a K07 Academic Award to the University of Pennsylvania School of Medicine for the development of our Cultural Competency Medical Education Program and the cases in this book.

Dr. Horace DeLisser would like to thank his wife, Opal, for her ongoing love, patience, and support throughout his professional career. He would also like to thank his parents, Oswald and Eileen, for their love and his sons, Horace Jr. and Jason, for all they have done to make their parents proud.

Dr. Lisa Hark would like to thank her children, Jamie and Brett, for their loving support and inspiration. She would also like to thank her parents, Diane and Jerry, for being the best parents anyone could ever have.

Both Drs. DeLisser and Hark dedicate this book to all the patients who have taught them the importance of listening better and how their cultural backgrounds influence so many issues related to medical care.

Introduction

Olivia Carter-Pakras, PhD and Horace DeLisser, MD

The importance of cultural competency

Over the last 50 years, increased non-European immigration, globalization, changing sexual norms, and the aging of the American population have resulted in a much more culturally diverse country with respect to race, ethnicity, age, religion, sexual identity and orientation, and beliefs about illness and health. As a result, health care providers are likely to encounter patients who will be culturally different from them. These cultural differences affect both patients' and providers' health beliefs, practices, and behaviors and influence their expectations of each other. Lack of awareness about cultural differences can make it difficult to achieve high-quality care. Miscommunication may result, and the provider may fail to understand why the patient does not follow instructions. For example, why the patient takes a smaller dose of a prescribed medicine (because of a belief that Western medicine is "too strong"); or why the family, rather than the patient, makes important decisions about the patient's health care (because major decisions are made by the family as a group in the patient's culture). Likewise, the patient may reject the provider (and the entire U.S. medical system) even before any one-on-one interaction occurs because of nonverbal cues that do not fit expectations.

Thus in the context of the provider–patient relationship, *cultural competence* refers to the health care provider's ability to work effectively with individuals from different cultural and ethnic backgrounds. Despite our similarities, fundamental differences among people arise from nationality, ethnicity, and culture, as well as from family background and individual experiences. *Cultural competency* refers to the ability to understand the language, culture, and behaviors of other individuals and groups, and to make appropriate recommendations. It also includes an awareness of one's own cultural influences as well as personal biases and prejudices. Cultural competency has been described as a "set of congruent behaviors, attitudes, and policies that come together in a system, agency or profession that enables that system, agency or profession to work effectively in cross-cultural situations" (1). This definition of cultural competency identifies systems, agencies, or professions as potential points of intervention. However, other definitions of cultural competency primarily address individuals *within* systems and pay less attention to other factors associated with social inequity.

Although varying definitions of culture exist, what is common to these definitions is the view that culture is a set of shared values, beliefs, patterns, and communication styles that characterize the social life of a group or society (1–11). Importantly, culture is not a static entity but rather a fluid and ever-changing set of values, knowledge, and beliefs and a learned behavior. By acknowledging, recognizing, and accounting for cultural issues, health care providers can deliver effective and appropriate care for patients in a variety of inpatient and outpatient settings.

Cultural sensitivity, which is a necessary component of cultural competence, means that health care professionals make an effort to be aware of the potential and actual cultural factors that affect their interactions with patients. It also means that they are willing to design and implement culturally relevant and specific programs and materials and to make related recommendations. The terms *cultural competence* and *culturally effective health care* are sometimes used synonymously.

Health disparities

Cultural competence has implications beyond the individual provider–patient relationship. Despite steady improvements in the overall health of the U.S. population, racial and ethnic minorities as a whole continue to experience disproportionately higher morbidity and mortality rates than nonminorities. For example, African Americans and Hispanic Americans (and to a less well-documented extent, Native American, Alaska Natives, Asian Americans, Native Hawaiians, and other Pacific Islanders) receive less medical care in general and fewer intensive care procedures compared to white patients (12–14). This pattern has been found in the use of high-technology interventions, such as angioplasty and coronary artery bypass surgery, and for medical and surgical procedures as well as the treatment of chronic conditions, such as diabetes. Men have higher prevalence of coronary heart disease, yet women die at higher rates. African American women have lower prevalence of breast cancer, yet die at higher rates. The reasons for these racial and ethnic disparities are complex and include multiple interconnected social and economic factors (12–15). In contributing to the elimination of these disparities, health professional students and providers must understand the underlying forces driving and maintaining these health disparities.

Differences in access to health care and differences in the quality of care received unquestionably contribute to health disparities. Timely use of personal health services to achieve the best health outcomes or health care access can be measured by (a) entry into the health care system, (b) structural barriers (e.g., transportation, ability to schedule appointments, and specialist referrals), (c) patient perceptions (e.g., patient–provider communication and relationships, cultural competency, health literacy, and health information), and (d) health care utilization (i.e., routine, acute, and chronic care, and avoidable hospital admissions).

While explanatory models for health disparities acknowledge the role of socioeconomic factors, they often include "culture" as a separate but related underlying factor (16–17). Freeman suggests that "poverty is reflected through the prism of culture . . . culture may augment or diminish poverty's expected effects" (16). Poverty or social and economic location within a society, combined with geopolitical context, shapes a racial, ethnic, or cultural group's access to social resources such as health care access and quality. Several views have been proposed on the role of culture in explaining health disparities. Some consider culture as a central or a significant predictor of health; some view it as having some role that is not yet clear, and others view it as a contextual variable that may promote or enhance the use of health services (18–25).

Although the National Healthcare Disparities Report does not specifically mention the role of bias and stereotyping, racial and ethnic bias and stereotyping by health care providers are thought to make significant contributions to health care disparities (12–14). Cultural competency training at all levels of professional education can play an important role in addressing racial and ethnic bias and stereotyping by health care providers.

Medical education

Cultural competence is now recognized by various governmental and accreditation agencies as essential for improving patients' health status and access to health care and for eliminating disparities in health care delivery. Health care system interventions to increase cultural competence can include programs to recruit and retain staff who reflect the cultural diversity of the community, use of interpreter services or bilingual providers, cultural competency training for health care providers, use of linguistically and culturally appropriate health education materials, and culturally specific health care settings (23). Health may be improved through these approaches because patients gain trust and confidence in accessing health care, and health care providers increase their ability to understand and treat a culturally diverse clientele. The effectiveness of these interventions can be assessed through intermediate outcomes and health outcomes. Examples of professional, governmental, and accrediting organizations recognizing the importance of cultural competency include the following:

(1) Association of American Medical Colleges (AAMC) Liaison Committee on Medical Education (LCME). Standards for accreditation of medical education programs leading to a medical degree in the U.S. and Canada require that medical students and faculty demonstrate an understanding of the manner in which people of diverse cultures and belief systems perceive health and illness and respond to various symptoms, diseases, and treatments (26). Medical schools are now required to document development of skills in cultural competence, indicate where in the curriculum students are exposed to such material, and demonstrate the extent to which the objectives are being achieved. Medical school instruction must stress the need for students to be concerned with the total medical needs of their patients and the effects that social and cultural circumstances have on their health. Clinical instruction is to include demographic influences on health care quality and effectiveness, such as racial and ethnic disparities in the diagnosis and treatment of diseases. Most importantly, self-awareness among students regarding any personal biases in their approach to health care delivery is to be addressed. The AAMC's recently published *Tool for Assessing Cultural Competence Training* (TACCT) is a comprehensive guide of objectives for the development of cultural competency and health disparities curriculum for undergraduate and graduate medical education (27, 28) and is shown in the introduction and Appendix 3.

(2) Accreditation Council for Graduate Medical Education (ACGME). In 1999, ACGME identified six core competencies for physicians: patient care, medical knowledge, practice-based learning and improvement, interpersonal and communication skills, professionalism, and systems-based practice (29). The fourth competency requires interpersonal and communication skills resulting in effective information exchange and collaboration with patients, their families, and other health professionals. The fifth competency, professionalism, includes "sensitivity to a diverse patient population." Health care organizations and health professional training programs are therefore beginning to develop cultural competence initiatives. Many organizations are getting social and legal pressures to do this from different segments of the population.

(3) The Department of Health and Human Services' Office of Minority Health. In 2001, the Office of Minority Health released the *National Standards for Culturally and Linguistically Appropriate Services in Health Care* (CLAS Standards) to guide health care organizations and individual providers in providing culturally effective health care (30).

(4) State Cultural Competency Training requirements. In 2005, New Jersey became the first state to require cultural competency training for physicians as a condition of licensure. More recently, Washington, California, New Mexico, and Maryland have passed legislation mandating or strongly recommending cultural competency training. A number of states are considering similar legislation (see http://www.thinkculturalhealth.org/cc_legislation.asp for a current update).

Using this book

Individuals working with different ethnic and cultural groups can become more culturally competent by advancing through three main stages: developing awareness, acquiring knowledge, and developing and maintaining cross-cultural communication and negotiation skills. *Achieving Cultural Competency: A Case-Based Approach to Training Health Professionals* is self-instructional, with case vignettes and questions, followed by case discussions. Twenty-five cases are presented in the areas of general medicine, cardiology, pulmonary medicine, hematology/oncology, neurology, pediatrics, endocrinology, and obstetrics and gynecology. Learners will not only gain knowledge, but have direct insight into real-life scenarios that have occurred in clinical settings.

The cases focus on how age, gender, socioeconomic position, race/ethnicity, sexual orientation, immigrant status, language, religious and spiritual practices, and folk beliefs and practices can affect the doctor–patient relationship. For example, the age of the patient may influence how the patient uses his/her time with the physician and/or how the patient is perceived by the physician (*Case 21*). Patients who are very young or very old may require the assistance of others in obtaining information and providing care (*Case 10*). The doctor–patient relationship may be negatively affected when the physician makes superficial judgments about patients based on stereotypes of a racial, ethnic, or socioeconomic (*Cases 2, 11, 24, 25*). A lack of patient empowerment, as a response to perceived higher status of the physician, may pose a barrier to building rapport, and result in an inability to question the physician's recommendations, or an overly trusting, dependent patient. A patient's perceptions of entitlement (i.e., deserving of special treatment), and whether the patient is rich or poor, can also negatively affect the doctor–patient relationship.

Ability to pay is considered the leading barrier to accessing health care. Financial constraints may result in poor health care due to lack of preventive care and/or later presentation for care. A patient may lack a primary care physician, be unable to pay for appropriate diagnostic tests and treatments (e.g., prescription medications), and/or depend on unreliable or expensive sources of transportation (*Case 2*). The daily experience with poverty, partner violence, drug use, poor housing, prostitution, and toxic environments impact not only the access to care, but also the patient's ability to prevent disease and its complications.

A patient's health literacy, associated either with low educational attainment or with a lack of understanding of health issues, can negatively affect the patient's ability to understand a diagnosis or participate as an active partner in developing and carrying out a treatment plan (*Case 9*). Health literacy can be unassociated with overall literacy and should be explored with all patients. Lack of reliable information (whether due to lack of money to pay for it, or lack of education to know whether and how to use it) can lead to an inability to understand or put into action the information provided. Individuals without ready access to a computer, or education or knowledge on how to use resources available at a library, may find it difficult to obtain needed information about self-care, illness, treatment, and resources.

Patients of the opposite gender as their physician may not feel comfortable discussing issues related to sexuality or sexual dysfunction. Gender discordance between the patient and the provider may affect the physician's ability to take a sensitive and thorough sexual history, and patients may prefer the same gender for OB/GYN and urology providers (*Cases 4, 13*). Gender bias in diagnosis and treatment may result in underconsideration of heart disease with females, overuse of cardiac catheterization with males, or presumption of males as perpetrators of partner violence and abuse (*Cases 17, 21*).

Stigma and the potential for discrimination serve as obstacles for lesbians and gays seeking appropriate health care (*Cases 8, 12*). Screening for interpartner violence with gay and lesbian patients is often overlooked and unattended. Establishing comfort and trust between the patient and the physician (i.e., the physician conveys and the patient feels that it is safe to disclose sexual orientation and sexual practices) is key to good doctor–patient communication.

Individual worldviews and belief systems (i.e., the meaning and significance of illness) of patients and physicians are shaped by the cultures in which they were raised and currently reside (*Cases 3, 5, 7, 13, 15, 20, 22*). Issues of trust/distrust due to historic racism (e.g., Tuskegee Study) and intergroup conflicts can negatively affect the doctor–patient relationship (*Cases 1, 16*). Racism on the part of the patient or physician may diminish the physician's ability to gather and/or interpret information about the patient and assure effective treatment and management (*Cases 1, 19*). For example, a young black man or woman presenting to the emergency department with pain while in a sickle cell crisis may be presumed to be a drug seeker (*Case 22*). Communication and interpersonal styles of communication that differ by culture may contribute to misunderstanding, misdiagnosis, or failure to develop rapport (*Cases 7, 23*). Values and traditions that conflict with mainstream "American" practices (e.g., female genital mutilation, objecting to an evaluation by provider of the opposite gender due to social norms, providing proof of virginity, seeking alternative therapies, and using euphemism to describe a terminal diagnosis) may affect the doctor–patient relationship.

Some of the meaning and significance of illness is shaped by the religious or spiritual traditions in which patients or their physicians are raised and/or currently practice (e.g., how a patient and family respond to death and dying) (*Cases 10, 14, 17*). Patient values and traditions stemming from religious/spiritual beliefs may conflict with those of their physician or health care system (e.g., end-of-life decisions, abortion, organ donation, and therapeutic practices such as use of blood products). Physician comfort and willingness to cooperate with certain patient practices can enhance the ability of the physician to establish rapport and build trust with the patient (e.g., patient's unwillingness to disrobe for physical examination, or patient's request to participate in or condone religious/spiritual practices such as asking the physician to pray with them) (*Case 25*). Some beliefs or practices may require or prohibit certain behaviors that can affect the patient's health or treatment (e.g., the challenge for diabetics of fasting during the Muslim holiday of Ramadan) (*Case 4*).

Verbal and nonverbal language differences between patients (and their families) and caregivers can diminish their ability to acquire accurate and timely information and provide care. Professional medical interpretation is needed in all places of care delivery since patients who speak English as a second language may not fully comprehend interviews or instructions in English (*Cases 6, 10, 11, 23*). Nonverbal language is also culturally based communication: assumptions cannot be made regarding the meanings attached to familiar actions (e.g., proximity, body language, gestures, and eye contact) (*Case 22*).

Patients may question the competence of foreign-born (immigrant) physicians or other health care providers due to pronounced accents, differences in cultures, and educational systems perceived as inferior (*Case 19*). The doctor–patient relationship may also be challenged by the expectations and experiences an immigrant patient brings to the encounter, and by the level of understanding and comfort the immigrant has of American culture (e.g., patients' lack of empowerment in the country of origin and concerns for safety especially with health care providers) (*Cases 6, 22*). The reason for immigration (e.g., economic opportunity or refugee status) and immigrant status may play important roles in the ability to access needed services. Immigrants who are living with undocumented family members, or who are undocumented themselves, delay presentation of symptoms and use fewer medical services (*Case 23*). Many immigrants work for smaller employers who do not provide paid leaves to attend medical appointments. Employment as seasonal workers can also prevent continuity of care and/or compliance with treatment. Given these issues, it is not surprising that the average lifespan of a male immigrant agricultural worker is 47 years as compared to a comparable white male.

Conclusion

In summary, health professionals in training and practice have been and will continue to be challenged to take care of patients and their families from many different ethnic and cultural groups who may live in the U.S. on a full- or part-time basis. Developing skills in cultural competency is an evolving process and it takes time, experience, and a commitment to listening and respecting patients and, above all, appreciating their perspective. It is our hope that *Achieving Cultural Competency: A Case-Based Approach to Training Health Professionals* will help with this process. Developed by a multidisciplinary team of medical educators experienced in cultural competency and health disparities education of medical students, physicians, and other health care professionals, this book of cases is the first of its kind.

Olivia Carter-Pokras, PhD
University of Maryland School of Public Health
College Park, MD, USA
Horace DeLisser, MD
University of Pennsylvania School of Medicine
Philadelphia, PA, USA

References

1. Cross T., Bazron B., Dennis K., Isaacs M. *Towards a Culturally Competent System of Care*, vol I. Georgetown University Child Development Center, CASSP Technical Assistance Center, Washington, DC, 1998.
2. Geertz C. *The Interpretation of Cultures: Selected Essays*. New York, Basic Books, 1973.
3. Merriam-Webster I. *Merriam-Webster's Medical Desk Dictionary*. Merriam-Webster Inc, Springfield, Mass, 2005.
4. Stedman T.L. *Stedman's Medical Dictionary*. Lippincott Williams & Wilkins, Philadelphia, 2006.
5. American Psychological Association. *Guidelines on Multicultural Education, Training, Research Practice and Organizational Change for Psychologists*. American Psychological Association, Washington, DC, 2002.
6. VandenBos G.R. *APA Dictionary of Psychology*. American Psychological Association, Washington, DC, 2007.
7. Last J.M. *A Dictionary of Public Health*. Oxford University Press, Oxford, 2007.
8. Giddens A. *Sociology*, 2nd edn. Polity Press, Oxford, 1993.

9. Schaefer R.T. *Sociology: A Brief Introduction*, 4th edn. McGraw-Hill, New York, 2002.

10. Johnson A.G. *The Blackwell Dictionary of Sociology: A User's Guide to Sociological Language*. Blackwell Publishers, Malden, Mass, 2000.

11. Winthrop R.H. *Dictionary of Concepts in Cultural Anthropology*. Greenwood Press, New York, 1991.

12. Physicians for Human Rights. *The Right to Equal Treatment: An Action Plan to End Racial and Ethnic Disparities in Clinical Diagnosis and Treatment in the United States*. Physicians for Human Rights, Cambridge, Mass, 2003.

13. Institute of Medicine. *Unequal Treatment: Confronting Racial and Ethnic Disparities in Health Care*. National Academies Press, Washington, DC, 2003.

14. Agency for Healthcare Research and Quality. *National Healthcare Disparities Report*. Agency for Healthcare Research and Quality, Washington, DC, 2006.

15. Carter-Pokras O., Baquet C. What is a health disparity? *Public Health Rep* 2002;117:426–32.

16. Freeman H. Commentary on the meaning of race in science and society. *Cancer Epidemiol Biomarkers Prev* 2003;12:232S–36S.

17. Brunner E., Marmot M. Social organization, stress, and health. In: Marmot M. & Wilkinson R.G., eds. *Social Determinants of Health*. Oxford University Press, New York, 1999.

18. Brach C., Fraser I. Can cultural competency reduce racial and ethnic health disparities? A review and conceptual model. *Med Care Res Rev* 2000;57:181–2 (suppl 1).

19. Johnson R.L., Somnath S., Arbelaez J., Beach M.C., Cooper L.A. Racial and ethnic differences in patient perceptions of bias and cultural competence in health care. *J Gen Intern Med* 2004;19:101–10.

20. Organista K.C. *Solving Latino Psychosocial and Health Problems*. John Wiley & Sons, Inc, Hoboken, NJ, 2007.

21. Collins F.S. What we do and don't know about "race," "ethnicity" genetics and health at the dawn of the genome era. *Nat Genet* 2004;36(11): S13–15.

22. Viruell-Fuentes E.A. Beyond acculturation: immigration, discrimination, and health research among Mexicans in the United States. *Soc Sci Med* 2007;65:1524–35.

23. Anderson L.M., Scrimshaw S.C., Fullilove M.T., Fielding J.E., Normand J. Culturally competent healthcare systems: a systematic review. *Am J Prev Med* 2003;24(3S):68–79.

24. Betancourt J.R., Green A.R., Carrillo E. *Cultural Competence in Health Care: Emerging Frameworks and Practical Approaches*. The Commonwealth Fund, New York, 2002.

25. Freimuth V., Quinn S. The contributions of health communication to eliminating health disparities. *Am J Pub Health* 2004;94(12): 2053–5.

26. Liaison Committee on Medical Education. *Functions and Structure of a Medical School: Standards for Accreditation of Medical Education Programs Leading to the M.D. Degree.* Association of American Medical Colleges, Washington, DC.

27. Association of American Medical Colleges. Tool for Assessing Cultural Competence Training (TACCT). Washington, DC. Available at: http://www.aamc.org/meded/tacct/start.htm.

28. Lie D.A., Boker J., Crandall S., DeGannes CN., Elliott D., MD, Henderson P., Kodjo C., and Seng L. Revising the Tool for Assessing Cultural Competence Training (TACCT) for curriculum evaluation: Findings derived from seven US schools and expert consensus.' *Med Educ Online.* 2008;13:11. Available at http://www.med-ed-online.org

29. Accreditation Council for Graduate Medical Education (ACGME) Outcome Project. General Competencies: Minimum Program Requirements Language, 1999. Available at: http://www.acgme.org.

30. Office of Minority Health. National Standards for Culturally and Linguistically Appropriate Services in Health Care (CLAS Standards). U.S. Department of Health and Human Services, Washington, DC, 2001. Available at: http://www.omhrc.gov.

Tools to Assess Cultural Competency Training (TACCT)	DOMAIN 1: Health Disparities	DOMAIN 2: Community Strategies	DOMAIN 3: Bias/Stereotyping	DOMAIN 4 : Communication skills specific to cross-cultural communication	DOMAIN 5: Use of Interpreters	DOMAIN 6: Self-reflection, culture of medicine
Introduction	x	x	x	x	x	x
Case 1: Ruth Franklin	x		x			x
Case 2: Carl Jones	x		x	x		
Case 3: Maria Morales	x	x		x		
Case 4: Maya Mohammad		x	x	x		
Case 5: Jon Lee	x		x	x		x
Case 6: Nadia Rosenberg				x	x	
Case 7: Isabel Delgado				x		x
Case 8: George Dennis			x			x
Case 9: Mary Jones	x			x		
Case 10: Priya Krishnamurthy		x		x	x	x
Case 11: Carlos Cruz				x	x	
Case 12: Denise Smith	x	x		x		x
Case 13: Mae Ling	x	x	x	x		
Case 14: Earl Collins				x		
Case 15: Irma Matos	x	x		x		
Case 16: Eileen Clark	x		x	x		
Case 17: Leslie O'Malley			x	x		x
Case 18: Juana Caban		x	x	x		x
Case 19: Alice Gregory	x		x	x		x
Case 20: Sulip Guha	x	x		x		
Case 21: Pepper Hawthorne	x		x	x		x
Case 22: Alika Nkuutu			x	x	x	
Case 23: Miguel Cortez				x	x	x
Case 24: Naomi Fulton	x	x		x		
Case 25: Bobby Napier		x	x	x		x

Source: Association of American Medical Colleges. Cultural Competence Education for Medical Students, Washington, DC. Available at: http://www.aamc.org/meded/tacct/start.htm

CASE 1

Ruth Franklin

A 40-year-old African American woman with heart failure

Susan E. Wiegers, MD and Horace DeLisser, MD
University of Pennsylvania School of Medicine, Philadelphia, PA, USA

Educational Objectives

- Explain how perceived racial differences and stereotyping by physicians may impact the patient–physician relationship.
- Review the health-related issues such as obesity that may be viewed differently by various racial and ethnic groups.
- Identify several factors that may lead to poor adherence to prescribed medications.
- Describe an approach for engaging a colleague whose behavior demonstrates cultural insensitivity.

TACCT Domains: 1, 3, 6

Case Summary, Questions and Answers

Mrs. Franklin is a 40-year-old African American woman who came to see Dr. Cox, a cardiologist, for management of congestive heart failure. She had seen another cardiologist in the group (Dr. Moore) 3 months earlier who had told her, "There is nothing wrong with you that losing 50 pounds won't cure." [She is 5'4" and weighs 235 lbs (BMI = 40) and has been overweight for all of her life.] This comment greatly angered Mrs. Franklin and so she did not follow-up with Dr. Moore.

Achieving Cultural Competency: A case-based approach to training health professionals,
1st edition. Edited by L Hark, H DeLisser. © 2009 Blackwell Publishing,
ISBN: 9781405180726.

1 What factors may have contributed to Mrs. Franklin's anger?

The insensitivity of Dr. Moore would certainly have provided sufficient reason for Mrs. Franklin to be angry. Clearly, it would have been better if Dr. Moore had addressed her need for weight loss in a more tactful and thoughtful way. However, it is important to recognize that Mrs. Franklin's past experiences with the health care system as an African American may shape the significance she might ascribe to Dr. Moore's comments and the intensity of her reaction. That is, Dr. Moore's comments are seen not as the mere words of a tactless individual, but are taken as another clear expression of a system that is hostile to African Americans. For Mrs. Franklin, the physician's behavior becomes part of a list of racially motivated mistreatments (real or perceived) she has experienced that are carried forward into her relationships with other physicians.

Rates of overweight and obesity are higher in African American and Hispanic females compared with other racial or ethnic groups, due to still incompletely understood interactions of genetic and/or environmental factors. Research suggests that minority women may be more accepting of larger body frames, more satisfied with their bodies, and less likely to perceive themselves as overweight. Further, when weight loss is attempted, African American women are less likely to have success. Thus, as an African American, the issue of weight loss for Mrs. Franklin may be one that involves ambivalence and/or past failures at managing her weight.

Consequently, understanding the nature of Mrs. Franklin's anger (*is it just about the insensitivity of Dr. Moore, or is there more?*) and then responding to it are essential for Dr. Cox to establish her relationship with the patient.

2 How should Dr. Cox address Mrs. Franklin's anger about her colleague?

The importance to the patient–physician relationship of addressing the patient's anger cannot be overstated. Mrs. Franklin's anger potentially interferes with her ability to listen effectively and may undermine trust and confidence in the recommendations and care of the physician. Further, her anger may be used to control the encounter and to prevent Dr. Cox from pursuing questions or issues that the patient may be uncomfortable answering. Conversely, making the effort to effectively respond to her anger provides a powerful message of respect that enhances the physician's alliance with the patient. Although the response should ultimately be individualized for each patient, it should be done in as nonconfrontational a way as possible using open-ended questions. Suggested questions include:

- *It is clear that what was said was very upsetting to you. Why did this make you so angry?*
- *What do you think motivated him to make this kind of comment?*
- *Given this experience, what concerns do you have about how I might treat you?*

> Over the past two years Mrs. Franklin has developed progressive dyspnea on exertion, and now has severe exercise intolerance. In addition, for the past 8 months, she has had increasing pedal edema, which is now severe and has resulted in venous stasis ulceration of her right leg. This is quite painful and she is also seeing an internist at the health clinic. In addition to a diuretic (furosimide), Mrs. Franklin had been prescribed an angiotensin receptor blocker (valsartan) but did not fill the prescription.

3   What additional information would be helpful in understanding why Mrs. Franklin did not fill her prescription?

A number of factors may influence the level of patient adherence to prescribed medications, recommended treatments, or health-promotion activities. These include life responsibilities, familial commitments, employment obligations, the level of financial resources, the quality of health insurance, as well as the psychological and emotional distractions resulting from these factors. The ability to pay for not only health insurance, but co-pays and deductibles, has been shown to be an important barrier. Also important are folk beliefs and the patient's understanding of his/her disease or illness. As she interviewed the patient, Dr. Cox learned that Mrs. Franklin is divorced with three children, 8- and 21-year-old daughters who live at home and a 19-year-old son who is away in the military. She is a manager at a convenience store and has employer-provided health insurance, but her plan does not cover prescription medications, such as valsartan. In the past 2 months, she has missed several days of work because of severe pain associated with her venous stasis ulcer. She has therefore been fearful of losing her job and her health insurance. Mrs. Franklin was not prescribed a more appropriate and less-expensive ACE inhibitor, but instead was prescribed a more expensive substitute. This may have been due to pharmaceutical samples that influenced the doctor to give these out. However, the ultimate consequence of her receiving these samples is that she is prescribed a medication that costs much more than other appropriate generic medications and she decides not to get it filled.

> *Medical therapy for congestive heart failure was subsequently begun with furosimide, spironolactone, enalapril, and metoprolol. Over the next 4 months, her blood pressure normalized and the pedal edema improved slightly, but there was no significant change in her dyspnea on exertion. During this time, she missed five of seven scheduled clinic visits without calling to cancel the visit, but she would call complaining of continued symptoms. For the two appointments Mrs. Franklin did keep, she was noted to be "hostile" and "distant." Dr. Cox did not confront Mrs. Franklin over these behaviors.*

4   How could Dr. Cox address missed clinic visits?

"Assuming" rather than "asking" is not necessarily respectful or culturally sensitive. The challenge is to be understanding, accommodating, and supportive without enabling behaviors and actions that are detrimental to the patient's care or health. In the patient–physician relationship, both sides have responsibilities. Failure by the physician to address self-defeating behaviors on the part of the patient ultimately undermines that relationship.

> *Six months after her initial office visit, Mrs. Franklin was admitted for worsening congestive heart failure. Dr. Cox suspected that Mrs. Franklin may not have been adherent in taking her medications but was also concerned that her underlying cardiomyopathy had progressed further. Dr. Biali was therefore consulted for cardiac transplant evaluation and for specialized heart failure care. The following day when Dr. Cox entered Mrs. Franklin's room, Mrs. Franklin angrily told her that she*

wanted to be discharged from the hospital and that under no circumstances should Dr. Biali be allowed in the room. She reported that Dr. Biali had criticized her for not taking her medications and for being overweight. He told her that she was not a transplant candidate unless she lost 100 lbs. Mrs. Franklin was incensed over Dr. Biali's approach and attitude.

5   How should Dr. Cox respond to Mrs. Franklin?

Dr. Cox faces the potentially difficult task of reestablishing the relationship in a way that does not dismiss or trivialize the emotion and pain of the patient, but still addresses appropriate concerns of the consultant. To that end it is important to not immediately take sides before first hearing from everyone involved. An initial comment of, *"What a terrible thing for Dr. Biali to say"* or *"There is no way Dr. Biali could say something like that,"* would not be helpful. Further, as noted above, it is important to recognize that the intensity of the patient's anger may reflect past negative experiences and/or culturally based perceptions or understandings of obesity. Dr. Cox should therefore first listen to Mrs. Franklin, respectfully acknowledging her emotions and then promise to speak with her again after meeting with Dr. Biali, hopefully presenting a plan with reasonable and achievable goals.

Cardiac Transplantation

Cardiac transplantation is the treatment of choice for selected patients with end-stage heart failure who remain significantly compromised despite optimal medical therapy. This has been made possible by the improvements in recipient and donor selection, advances in immunosuppression, and prevention and treatment of infection. Currently, there is a 15% to 20% mortality in the first year, with a mortality rate of about 3.4% per year thereafter. The major causes of death are acute allograft rejection, infections (other than cytomegalovirus), allograft vasculopathy, and lymphoma and malignancies.

Although more than 4000 cardiac transplants are performed worldwide each year, there continues to be a chronic and severe shortage of available donor hearts. As a result, recipient selection and donor allocation are significant clinical and ethical issues.

> Dr. Cox went to speak to Dr. Biali about the interaction. Dr. Biali noted that the patient had admitted to him that she intermittently used cocaine and in his judgment was not a transplant candidate. He said flatly, "Your patient is a dirtball with cocaine cardiomyopathy and I'll transplant her over my dead body." [Dr. Biali is the only transplant cardiologist at the hospital. He is the only person who can list the patient for transplant, and there is no other transplant program in this city.]

6   Is Dr. Biali just using colorful language, or does his choice of words reflect a bias or prejudice? If so, what might that bias or prejudice be?

In most instances, we can never know with absolute certainty what motivates an individual's behavior. However, the use of the word "dirtball" (a very pejorative phrase), reference to "cocaine cardiomyopathy" (a questionable entity), and insistence of a 100-lb weight loss (an arbitrary requirement) all raise concern about Dr. Biali's attitudes and motivation. His possible biases include not only race, but also class and socioeconomic status, along with the clash between the lay culture and the culture of medicine.

7   How should Dr. Cox approach Dr. Biali regarding his perception of Mrs. Franklin?

In a respectful but professional way, Dr. Cox should directly discuss with Dr. Biali her concerns regarding his behavior, while acknowledging the need to be a good steward of a scarce resource. Ultimately, she needs to continue to be an advocate for the patient, working to establish achievable goals that appropriately address Dr. Biali's concerns (e.g. 6 months of negative random drug screens, 20-lb weight loss, compliance with office visits). Unwillingness on the part of Dr. Biali to cooperate with Dr. Cox in developing a fair and appropriate plan for the patient may require mediation at a higher, institutional level.

Ethnic and Racial Disparities in Organ Transplantation

According to data collected by the United Network for Organ Sharing, there are currently more than 98,000 people in America who are waiting for organ donation. Nearly half of that list is comprised of people who identify themselves as non-Hispanic whites. More than a quarter

(27.2%) are black, 15.5% are Hispanic, 5% are Asian, 0.9% are American Indian/Alaska Native, 0.5% are Pacific Islander, and the remaining portion identify themselves as multiracial or unknown. The same data reveal that the ethnic make-up of the population who received transplant in 2006 was somewhat different, substantiating the claim that ethnic minorities are receiving fewer organ donations. For those patients who received a transplant in 2006, 62.7% were non-Hispanic whites, 18.9% were black, 12.3% were Hispanic, 4.1% were Asian, 0.8% were American Indian/Alaska Native, and 0.3% were Pacific Islander. Compared with their white counterparts, black and Hispanic patients encounter longer delays in getting referred, spend longer times on transplant waiting lists, and have lower rates of graft survival and higher mortality after receiving a transplanted organ.

The causes of these disparities are multiple, complex, and not fully understood. Biological processes that have been proposed to account for these observed racial and ethnic differences include greater variations in human leukocyte antigen polymorphisms, differences in immunosuppression requirements, and differences in the pharmacokinetics of immunosuppressive medications and immunologic responsiveness. A number of other nonbiological, sociocultural explanations have also been offered, including racism, socioeconomic status and class, unfavorable geographical location, lack of organ donation by minority groups, differences in social networks, culturally related health beliefs, and poorer control of hypertension in African Americans. Eliminating these disparities will prove to be challenging because the precise attributable disparity risk associated with the various factors is not known and many of the causes are tightly intertwined with each other.

References: Case 1

Briley C.A. Obesity among postpartum African-American adolescents. *J Am Dietetic Assoc* 2006;106:87–88.

Chakkera H.A., O'Hare A.M., Johansen K.L., et al. Influence of race on kidney transplant outcomes within and outside the Department of Veterans Affairs. *J Am Soc Nephrol* 2005;16:269–77.

Cheng J.W. A review of isosorbide dinitrate and hydralazine in the management of heart failure in black patients, with a focus on a new fixed-dose combination. *Clin Ther* 2006;28:666–78.

Churak J.M. Racial and ethnic disparities in renal transplantation. *J Natl Med Assoc* 2005;97:153–60.

Dans P.E. The use of pejorative terms to describe patients: "Dirtball" revisited. *Proc (Bayl Univ Med Cent)* 2002;15:26–30.

Davis E.M., Clark J.M., Carrese J.A., et al. Racial and socioeconomic differences in the weight-loss experiences of obese women. *Am J Public Health* 2005;95:1539–43.

Fallon E.M., Tanofsky-Kraff M., Norman A.C., et al. Health-related quality of life in overweight and non-overweight black and white adolescents. *J Pediatr* 2005;47:443–50.

Hunt S.A. American College of Cardiology; American Heart Association task force on practice guidelines (writing committee to update the 2001 guidelines for the evaluation and management of heart failure). ACC/AHA 2005 guideline update for the diagnosis and management of chronic heart failure in the adult. *J Am Coll Cardiol* 2005;46:e1–82.

James D.C. Gender differences in body mass index and weight loss strategies among African Americans. *J Am Diet Assoc* 2003;103:1360–2.

Kulkarni S.P., Alexander K.P., Lytle B., et al. Long-term adherence with cardiovascular drug regimens. *Am Heart J* 2006;151:185–91.

Kumanyika S. Obesity in black women. *Epidemiol Rev* 1987;29:31–50.

Kumanyika S.K., Morssink C., Agurs T. Models for dietary and weight change in African-American women: identifying cultural components. *Ethn Dis* 1992;2:166-75.

Lederer D.J., Caplan-Shaw C.E., O'Shea M.K., et al. Racial and ethnic disparities in survival in lung transplant candidates with idiopathic pulmonary fibrosis. *Am J Transplant* 2006;6:398–403.

Lunsford S.L., Simpson K.S., Chavin K.D., et al. Racial differences in coping with the need for kidney transplantation and willingness to ask for live organ donation. *Am J Kidney Dis* 2006;47:324–31.

Mahle W.T., Kanter K.R., Vincent R.N. Disparities in outcome for black patients after pediatric heart transplantation. *J Pediatr* 2005;147:739–43.

Moore D.E., Feurer I.D., Rodgers S. Jr, et al. Is there racial disparity in outcomes after solid organ transplantation? *Am J Surg* 2004;188:571–4.

Osterberg L., Blaschke T. Adherence to medication. *N Engl J Med* 2005; 353:487–97.

Peters T.G. Racial disparities and transplantation. *Am J Kidney Dis* 2005; 46:760–2.

Press R., Carrasquillo O., Nickolas T., Radhakrishnan J., Shea S., Barr R.G. Race/ethnicity, poverty status, and renal transplant outcomes. *Transplantation* 2005;80:917–24.

Poston R.S., Griffith B.P. Heart transplantation. *J Intensive Care Med* 2004; 19:3–12.

Shanewise J. Cardiac transplantation. *Anesthesiol Clin North Am* 2004;22:753–65.

Tang W.H., Francis G.S. The year in heart failure. *J Am Coll Cardiol* 2005; 46:2125–33.

Wong B.W., Rahmani M., Rezai N., McManus B.M. Progress in heart transplantation. *Cardiovasc Pathol* 2005;14:176–80.

White H.D. Adherence and outcomes: it's more than taking the pills. *Lancet* 2005;366:1989–91.

The Organ Procurement and Transplant Network (2006, June 16). Organ by ethnicity: current U.S. waiting list. Available at: http://www.optn.org/latestData/rptData.asp.

CASE 2

Carl Jones

A 48-year-old homeless Caucasian man with chest pain and lung cancer

Lisa Bellini, MD

University of Pennsylvania School of Medicine, Philadelphia, PA, USA

Educational Objectives

- Take into account that physicians may have biases related to socioeconomic status that may influence their clinical decisions and ultimately patient care.
- Discuss how patient homelessness impacts physician attitudes and disease management.
- Demonstrate the ways in which differences in socioeconomic status may affect patient–physician communication.

TACCT Domains: 1, 3, 4

Case Summary, Questions and Answers

Mr. Jones is a 48-year-old Caucasian military veteran who presents to the Emergency Department (ED) requesting analgesics for intermittent right-sided chest pain that he has been experiencing for the past week. He smokes one pack of cigarettes a day, but has no other risk factors for coronary artery disease. The remainder of his medical history is notable only for posttraumatic stress disorder and mild schizophrenia. Although

Achieving Cultural Competency: A case-based approach to training health professionals,
1st edition. Edited by L Hark, H DeLisser. © 2009 Blackwell Publishing,
ISBN: 9781405180726.

he has been through multiple substance abuse programs, he continues to use crack cocaine and alcohol daily. He is unemployed and homeless but receives a small stipend for military-related disabilities and has access to full medical care through the Veterans Administration. Mr. Jones appears disheveled and smells of alcohol, but his physical exam is otherwise unremarkable.

1 What issues does this patient encounter raise and what additional information might be helpful in caring for Mr. Jones?

Mr. Jones' low socioeconomic status (manifested by his homelessness and his lack of employment) is inextricably intertwined with his substance abuse and mental illness. In addition, a trauma history (from his military service) could be contributing to his behavior, mental health, and drug use. These factors, in turn, speak to his decision-making capacity and his ability to do those things required for his health, issues that will ultimately have an impact on any treatment plan.

Homelessness in the U.S.

A person is considered to be homeless if s/he lacks a fixed, regular, and adequate nighttime residence and has a primary nighttime residency that is: (a) a supervised publicly or privately operated shelter designed to provide temporary living accommodations; (b) a place that provides a temporary residence for individuals intended to be institutionalized; or (c) a public or private place not designed for, or ordinarily used as, a regular sleeping accommodation for human beings.

Over the course of a year, 2.3 to 3.5 million people will experience an episode of homelessness, with about 800,000 Americans sleeping on the street or in shelters each night. The homeless, however, represent a very diverse group, which includes families with children, single women, street youths between the ages of 15 and 24 years, and single men (the largest group). Although most people use homeless shelters for a period of only weeks to months before finding more permanent housing in the community, between 10% and 20% of shelter residents are chronically homeless. These individuals, for whom the shelters represent a semipermanent home, experience high rates of drug and alcohol addiction (see below).

The prevalence of physical disease, mental illness, and substance abuse is high among the homeless. Homelessness is also associated with exposure to the elements and an increased risk of infections, such as tuberculosis and human immunodeficiency virus (HIV) infection. Further, the homeless are burdened by poverty, typically have suboptimal access to health care, and often come from disadvantaged minority communities, factors that are independently associated with poor health. Thus, it is not surprising that mortality among homeless persons is much higher than among their counterparts in the general population.

While in the ED, an electrocardiogram (ECG) and chest x-ray are obtained and Mr. Jones is treated with aspirin, supplemental oxygen, and lorazepam. His ECG is normal and the pain resolved. An abnormality is also noted on his chest x-ray in the right lower lobe. He is discharged with a prescription for ibuprofen and given specific instructions to follow-up with his primary care provider (PCP) for further evaluation within 1 month.

2   Did Mr. Jones receive the "standard of care" for new-onset chest pain in the ED?

No, the standard of care would have been to admit Mr. Jones for evaluation of new-onset chest pain to rule out a myocardial infarction. Biases on the part of the ED staff could have contributed to the decision to discharge the patient rather than admit him for further cardiac workup. First, physicians are a privileged and advantaged group, and so even the most well-intentioned physician is not immune to socioeconomic and class biases. Second, self-destructive behaviors by patients (such as substance abuse) often trigger negative responses from health care providers. These may include frustration, and even a sense of futility, over caring for individuals who are not in control of their lives and whose behavior appears resistant to change. Providers may also feel anger over patients' misuse of governmental aid to support their negative behaviors. The key to minimizing the influence of these factors on physician judgment is to have physicians first acknowledge their own vulnerability to these biases, and then scrutinize their decisions to insure that they are not tainted by these biases. The question physicians should ask themselves is: *Would the treatment plan have been different if this patient were a financially well-off, employed, non–drug-using individual?*

3 Was it sufficient to assume that the patient was capable of achieving follow-up care on his own?

Given the entirety of his medical history, a strong argument could have been made for having a lower threshold for admitting Mr. Jones. This question, however, speaks more fundamentally to a tension between respecting the patient's autonomy, which includes allowing individuals to take responsibility for their heath, and a paternalism for "the good of the patient" that marginalizes the patient because he is poor, homeless, and abusing drugs.

Over the next month, Mr. Jones presented three times to the ED to obtain medication refills for chest and back pain. He was instructed on each occasion to follow-up with his PCP but did not do so. On at least one of these ED visits, he smelled of alcohol and was disrespectful to the staff. He was subsequently seen 7 months later at a free local clinic complaining of moderately severe chest and back pain, along with nasal congestion and cough. He was given ibuprofen and decongestants and instructed to see his doctor. He did, in fact, schedule an appointment for the following month but failed to keep it. Twelve months after his initial ED visit for chest pain, Mr. Jones again presented to the ED with a 3-week history of coughing up blood and "walking pneumonia." He was admitted after a chest x-ray revealed a large mass in his right lower lobe.

---

4 What barriers to adherence (compliance) are illustrated in this case?

The term adherence refers to the extent to which patients take medications as prescribed or follow the treatment regimens, instructions, or recommendations of their health care providers. Table 2.1 summarizes important barriers to adherence that exist, related to patients, physicians, or the health care system. Poor adherence may result in significant worsening of disease, death, and increased health care costs, which may or may not be related to a patient's socioeconomic status.

Table 2.1 Important patient, physician, and health care system barriers to adherence

Patient	Physician	Health care system
Presence of psychological problems (e.g. depression)	Poor doctor–patient relationship	Cost of medications or treatment
Presence of cognitive impairments	Prescribing complex treatments or regimens	Restrictive institutional formularies
Lack of belief in the need or benefit of treatment	Inadequate follow-up or discharge planning	Inadequate health insurance
Lack of insight into the illness	Inadequate explanations of instructions	High insurance copayment
Forgetfulness		
Distraction by other life issues or priorities (e.g. job, family)		
Medication side effects		
Treatment of asymptomatic disease		

Source: Lisa Bellini, MD, University of Pennsylvania School of Medicine. 2009. Used with permission.

5   If this patient were a lawyer and had missed several appointments because of conflicts with court dates but had called the office to have the pain medications renewed, should he have been treated differently?

It is hard to deny that wealth and prestige may enable certain advantages in the health care system, such as being able to call in repeatedly for prescription refills of analgesics without being properly evaluated. The challenge for the physician is to always provide care that is in the best interest of the patient and promotes the patient's health, regardless of the patient's status.

> *Mr. Jones' eventual hospital course included confirmation of a primary lung cancer with abdominal metastases, resulting in bowel necrosis and chronic gastrointestinal bleeding, which required almost daily blood transfusions. The medical team recommended a discharge from the hospital with palliative and hospice care, but Mr. Jones vigorously resisted changing the focus of his care to comfort measures only. As a result, he remained hospitalized while discussions continued with the patient about hospice care. Four weeks into his hospitalization, he sustained a cardiac arrest. Resuscitative efforts were attempted but were not successful.*

6 What role might the patient's low socioeconomic status have played in the recommendation of the team to pursue comfort care or the patient's resistance to this approach?

Given that Mr. Jones had end-stage metastatic cancer, efforts to advance his level of care to comfort measures were appropriate. However, the differences in class between physicians and patients may create barriers to communication and/or prevent physicians from being able to truly understand the patient's perspective.

Whereas conversations about changing the focus of care to comfort measures at the end of life may be seen by educated or more financially secure patients as positive efforts to respect autonomy, poor or disadvantaged individuals may instead view these discussions as an attempt to deny them essential treatments. Further, for a patient without a strong support network of family and friends and for whom "home" does not really exist, the opportunity to die outside of the hospital ("at home among family and friends") would not carry much appeal.

References: Case 2

Alter D.A., Iron K., Austin P.C., Naylor C.D. SESAMI Study Group. Socioeconomic status, service patterns, and perceptions of care among survivors of acute myocardial infarction in Canada. *JAMA* 2004;291:1100–7.

Bloom S.L. *Creating Sanctuary: Toward the Evolution of Sane Societies.* Routledge, New York, 1997.

Caton C.L., Dominguez B., Schanzer B., et al. Risk factors for long-term homelessness: findings from a longitudinal study of first-time homeless single adults. *Am J Public Health* 2005;95:1753–9.

Cheung A.M., Hwang S.W. Risk of death among homeless women: a cohort study and review of the literature. *Can Med Assoc J* 2004;170:1243–7.

Hwang S.W. Mortality among men using homeless shelters in Toronto, Ontario. *JAMA* 2000;283:2152–7.

Hwang S.W. Homelessness and health. *Can Med Assoc J* 2001;164:229–33.

Hwang S.W., Tolomiczenko G., Kouyoumdjian F.G., et al. Interventions to improve the health of the homeless: a systematic review. *Am J Prev Med* 2005;29:311–9.

Hwang S.W. Homelessness and harm reduction. *Can Med Assoc J* 2006;174: 50–1.

International Early Lung Cancer Action Program Investigators; Henschke C.I., Yankelevitz D.F., Libby D.M., et al. Survival of patients with stage I lung cancer detected on CT screening. *N Engl J Med* 2006;355:1763–71.

Jett J.R., Miller Y.E. Update in lung cancer 2005. *Am J Respir Crit Care Med* 2006;173:695–7.

Kulkarni S.P., Alexander K.P., Lytle B., Heiss G., Peterson E.D. Long-term adherence with cardiovascular drug regimens. *Am Heart J* 2006;151:185–91.

Kushel M.B., Miaskowski C. End-of-life care for homeless patients: "she says she is there to help me in any situation." *JAMA* 2006;296:2959–66.

Morris D.M., Gordon J.A. The role of the emergency department in the care of homeless and disadvantaged populations. *Emerg Med Clin North Am* 2006;24:839–48.

Osterberg L., Blaschke T. Adherence to medication. *N Engl J Med* 2005; 353:487–97.

Saijo N. Recent trends in the treatment of advanced lung cancer. *Cancer Sci* 2006;97:448–52.

Singh S.M., Paszat L.F., Li C., He J., Vinden C., Rabeneck L. Association of socioeconomic status and receipt of colorectal cancer investigations: a population-based retrospective cohort study. *Can Med Assoc J* 2004;171: 461–5.

Strauss G.M. Overview and clinical manifestations of lung cancer. UpToDate. Available at: http://www.utdol.com.

Sugimura H., Yang P. Long-term survivorship in lung cancer: a review. *Chest* 2006;129:1088–97.

Tedeschi R.G., Park C.L., Calhoun L.G. *Posttraumatic Growth: Positive Changes in the Aftermath of Crisis.* Lawrence Erlbaum Associates,, Mahwah, NJ, 1998.

White H.D. Adherence and outcomes: it's more than taking the pills. *Lancet* 2005;366:1989–91.

CASE 3

Maria Morales

A 57-year-old Mexican woman with type 2 diabetes

Desiree Lie, MD, MSEd,[1] *and Charles Vega, MD*[2]

[1]University of California at Irvine, Orange, CA, USA
[2]University of California at Irvine, Irving, CA, USA

Educational Objectives

- Describe the prevalence of type 2 diabetes among Latinos and other ethnic groups of patients.
- Identify some prevalent health beliefs associated with diabetes care and management among Latino patients.
- Report challenges and motivators associated with diabetes care in patients with different health beliefs.
- Describe strategies to seek resources for improving education and adherence among patients with type 2 diabetes from different cultural backgrounds.

TACCT Domains: 1, 2, 4

Case Summary, Questions and Answers

Mrs. Morales is a 57-year-old Mexican American woman who presents to her primary care physician (PCP), Dr. Morris, for follow-up of her type 2 diabetes and hypertension. She has had diabetes for 9 years, and her hemoglobin A1C level averages about 9.5% (normal <7.0%). Her current BMI is 33 kg/m², and she has gained 4 lbs

Achieving Cultural Competency: A case-based approach to training health professionals,
1st edition. Edited by L Hark, H DeLisser. © 2009 Blackwell Publishing,
ISBN: 9781405180726.

since her last visit 3 months ago. She is taking a sulfonylurea, a statin, and an ACE inhibitor. Mrs. Morales says to Dr. Morris, "I need to lose some weight. Can you help me? My family (2 adult children and 3 grandchildren, ages 2 to 6 years) are worried about me and they need me around." Dr. Morris hands her an American Diabetes Association 1800-calorie diet and tells her to eat less, add more fruits and vegetables, and exercise more to help control her diabetes, reinforcing what he has previously suggested over the years. She is scheduled to follow-up in 2 months.

1   Why has Dr. Morris' approach been ineffective in helping Mrs. Morales lose weight and reduce her A1c levels?

Nutritional management and lifestyle changes, in conjunction with prescribed medications, are the cornerstone of treatment for patients with type 2 diabetes. It is easy for Dr. Morris to suggest that she eat less and exercise more, but this recommendation is too vague for Mrs. Morales to implement, and does not factor in the influences of her traditional ethnic background. Effective dietary change requires specific suggestions that take into account a patient's food preferences, work and family schedule, and most importantly cultural heritage. Food plays an important role in most cultures, including Hispanic cultures. Many Latino families are more likely than other cultures to prepare and serve food at home, as well as to eat with the family. Research shows that Latino patients may also be more likely to change their eating habits if they receive a diagnosis of a health problem, physician advice to change diet, and/or are concerned for the health of their children or spouse.

2   What other information could Dr. Morris elicit to better understand Mrs. Morales' perception of her diabetes?

Most Latinos living in the U.S. recognize that diabetes is caused by negative health behaviors, such as poor diet and lack of exercise, as well as a family history of the disease. However, many patients may also believe that experiencing strong emotions, such as fright (*susto*), intense anger (*coraje*), or sadness and depression (*tristeza*), may also precipitate diabetes. Although the majority of Latino patients believe it is important to take oral medications and insulin as recommended by their doctor, they may also seek the advice of holistic healers (*curanderos*) to help treat their diabetes. Complementary and alternative medicine (CAM) treatments, such as prickly pear cactus (*nopal*) or aloe vera (*sevila*), may be used. Latino patients who aggressively seek alternative therapies are also more likely to seek traditional medical care and combine the two modalities in their personal treatment, as is true for most patients using CAM.

To reduce the risk of herb–drug interactions, a careful history should be taken to elicit the use of alternative medicine recommendations from *curanderos* or other family members. Being accepting of the patients' concerns and asking questions about alternative therapies in a nonjudgmental manner will help develop rapport with patients. Mrs. Morales admits to using herbal remedies and believes that they have helped her to feel better.

3   What role might Mrs. Morales' family play in helping her to improve her diet and lifestyle?

From Mrs. Morales' response, she is ready to make changes and is reaching out to Dr. Morris for help. Mrs. Morales has a strong sense of family and would like to remain healthy for herself, her husband, her children, and her grandchildren. This is a powerful motivator for her to engage in lifestyle changes to improve her diabetes outcomes. By encouraging her to bring a relative for future visits, Dr. Morris can explain the risks and recommended lifestyle changes for the family. Mrs. Morales is willing to involve her family, and this offer is likely to produce positive reinforcement of the physician's recommendations. Familial support appears to be critical to Latino patients' confidence in their ability to control diabetes, and men are more likely to receive support compared with women.

Prevalence of diabetes in Latino population

The prevalence of type 2 diabetes is 1.5 times higher in Latinos than non–Latino whites. Two million or 8.2% of all Latinos ages 20 years or older have diabetes. Approximately 24% of Mexican Americans, 26% of Puerto Ricans, and nearly 16% of Cuban Americans in the U.S. between the ages of 45 and 74 years have diabetes. The Centers for Disease Control and Prevention (CDC) and American Diabetes Association both highlight ethnic differences in the prevalence, treatment, and risks of diabetes.

> *Mrs. Morales returns for her 2-month follow-up appointment. Her weight has not changed, and Dr. Morris insists that she start exercising or she may have to go on insulin therapy to control her blood sugar and A1c level. Mrs. Morales responds by saying that insulin is not an option for her. She also says that she has been told by many doctors over the years that she should take up "somewhat strenuous exercise that makes her short of breath," such as running or bicycling, to benefit her heart and to prevent the bad outcomes of diabetes. However, she states that her daily housework, which includes vacuuming, cleaning the floors, cooking, gardening, and shopping for the family, is sufficient exercise and that she has no desire to start anything new at this stage in her life. Dr. Morris refers her to the dietitian working with his primary care practice. She is scheduled to follow-up again in 2 months. The next day, Mrs. Morales speaks to the dietitian on the phone, but does not make an appointment to see her.*

4   Why might Mrs. Morales have been reluctant to make an appointment with the dietitian after an initial conversation?

Referring Mrs. Morales to a dietitian for nutrition and lifestyle counseling was a positive step in her treatment. Working within a diabetes care team, which includes dietitians, nurses, social workers, podiatrists, psychologists, and exercise physiologists, has been shown to improve patient outcomes. Registered dietitians have the time and are trained in developing individualized diabetic diets and modifying traditional recipes based on the patient's personal food preferences. This nutrition counseling session could also encompass motivational interviewing to encourage her to begin a realistic exercise program and address the barriers that she describes regarding strenuous exercise and her shortness of breath.

However, when Mrs. Morales called and spoke with the dietitian, she found out that the dietitian did not speak Spanish. Mrs. Morales immediately concluded that the dietitian would not understand the dietary needs of her family and their Mexican diet. In order to ensure that Mrs. Morales would make and keep her appointment with the dietitian, the physician should have done the following:
- Recognized that this is not a routine nutrition referral for diabetes because of the potential ethnic and language issues;
- Discussed the importance of the referral with the patient;

- Explained that he will make an attempt to identify a bilingual dietitian; and
- Called the dietitian to familiarize her with the potential cultural and ethnic issues of this patient.

5 How can Dr. Morris best address Mrs. Morales' perceptions and fear of insulin therapy, and are there particular health beliefs that may impact Mrs. Morales' future diabetes care?

Most patients presenting to physicians' offices have a real interest in controlling their diabetes and adhering to medical treatment. Physicians should explore the beliefs of the patient regarding treatment of diabetes, which will vary by country of origin, personal experience, and educational level. Some Latino patients believe that the use of insulin causes blindness or renal damage. People holding this belief will therefore be more likely to resist insulin therapy. Too often, physicians use insulin as a threat: "if you don't take your pills, I will put you on insulin." This results in a lack of understanding of the nature of diabetes. Many patients with diabetes, as the disease progresses, require insulin, and this needs to be explained rather than using insulin as a threat. Mrs. Morales is not open to insulin therapy as she believes that the use of insulin could cause blindness, kidney failure, and a rapid decline in her health. She states that she has seen this happen to other people she knows who have diabetes. The casual nature of using insulin with progressively worsening disease, can be confusing to patients, and family stories reinforce this myth. Physicians need to clarify cause and effect.

Adherence to procedures to treat diabetes complications, such as retinopathy or renal disease, are generally well received. A full explanation of each procedure and potential complications, with the patient summarizing the information back to the physician, is highly recommended.

Mrs. Morales returns to the office 2 months later and admits to Dr. Morris that she did not make an appointment to see the dietitian. When asked why, Mrs. Morales says she had trouble understanding her on the phone. Dr. Morris realizes that a referral for a bilingual dietitian familiar with the Mexican diet would be helpful. Mrs. Morales agrees to see a Spanish-speaking dietitian. She then asks Dr. Morris whether her two children (ages 28 and 30 years) and her three grandchildren (ages 2 to 6 years) are at risk of getting diabetes and what, if anything, they can do to prevent diabetes. Dr. Morris gives her patient education materials in Spanish for herself and her family and directs her to a Spanish language Web site for people with diabetes.

6   What assumptions did Dr. Morris make in responding to Mrs. Morales' request regarding her family's risk of developing diabetes?

Studies show that U.S. Latinos are less likely to receive diabetes education compared with other ethnicities. Therefore, health professionals need to provide culturally appropriate information to this group in particular. Once Dr. Morris realized that she needed Spanish language materials and nutrition counseling, he provided recommendations. However, he assumed that she had a computer and could access the Internet and that she was literate in both English and Spanish. Unfortunately, none of the above was true for her. Mrs. Morales only completed primary school in Mexico and she does not read English. She does not have a computer in her home, but her children do and they have access to the Internet. Having family members help her access the information will give her the support she needs and educate her family as well, because they will most likely have to read the information to her.

Numerous resources are available to access the latest evidence-based guidelines for diabetes care. In recent years, the World Health Organization, the American Diabetes Association, and other organizations have revised the definitions of prediabetes and diabetes to lower (more stringent) blood glucose levels. The risk of metabolic syndrome associated with type 2 diabetes has been increasingly recognized. These changes are likely to result in greater numbers of patients being identified with diabetes and metabolic syndrome and the need for more aggressive management strategies to prevent type 2 diabetes. It is important to assist patients to identify sources of evidence-based advice, as many health-related Web sites are portals for commercial products. Examples of resources include:

- http://diabetes.niddk.nih.gov/index.htm. National Diabetes Information Clearinghouse (NDIC). Diabetes Overview *NIH Publication No. 04-3873, April 2004.*
- http://www.diabetes.org/about-diabetes.jsp. All About Diabetes – American Diabetes Association. (A good site to obtain background information about all areas of diabetes, including types, symptoms, risk test, statistics, prevention, etc.)

Mrs. Morales returns to see Dr. Morris 4 months later. She has seen the dietitian, initiated some dietary changes, and started walking 15 minutes on most days during the week. She has lost 5 lbs and plans to follow-up with the dietitian every few months. She states that she is willing to continue walking every day and following a healthy diet in order to avoid insulin injections. Dr. Morris congratulates Mrs. Morales on her weight loss and successful implementation of an exercise regimen. He explains that her hemoglobin A1c has now fallen to 8.0%, and this positive outcome is due to her lifestyle changes. He agrees not to begin an insulin regimen and to consider other means of improving her diabetes control, should the HbA1c not reach the desired level of 7.0% or lower.

References: Case 3

Alcozer F. Secondary analysis of perceptions and meanings of type 2 diabetes among Mexican-American women. *Diabetes Educ* 2000;26(5):785–95.

American Diabetes Association. Evidence-based nutrition principles and recommendations for the treatment and prevention of diabetes and related complications (Position Statement). *Diabetes Care* 2004;27:S55–7 (suppl 1).

Bertera E.M. Psychosocial factors and ethnic disparities in diabetes diagnosis and treatment among older adults. *Health Soc Work* 2003;28(1):33–42.

Black S.A., Markides K.S., Ray L.A. Depression predicts increased incidence of adverse health outcomes in older Mexican-Americans with type 2 diabetes. *Diabetes Care* 2003;26(10):2822–8.

Brown S.A., Becker H.A., Garcia A.A., Barton S.A., Hanis C.L. Measuring health beliefs in Spanish-speaking Mexican-Americans with type 2 diabetes: adapting an existing instrument. *Res Nurs Health* 2002;25(2):145–58.

Brown S.A., Harrist R.B. Gender and treatment differences in knowledge, health beliefs, and metabolic control in Mexican-Americans with type 2 diabetes. *Diabetes Educ* 2000;26(3):425–38.

Centers for Disease Control and Prevention (CDC). Prevalence of diabetes among Hispanics–selected areas, 1998-2002.*MMWR Morb Mortal Wkly Rep* 2004;53(40):941–4.

Chesla C.A., Skaff M.M., Bartz R.J., Mullan J.T., Fisher L. Differences in personal models among Latinos and European Americans: implications for clinical care. *Diabetes Care* 2000;23(12):1780–5.

Coronado G.D., Thompson B., Tejeda S., Godina R. Attitudes and beliefs among Mexican Americans about type 2 diabetes. *J Healthcare Poor Underserved* 2004;15(4):576–88.

Daniulaityte R. Making sense of diabetes: cultural models, gender and individual adjustment to type 2 diabetes in a Mexican community. *Soc Sci Med* 2004;59(9):1899–912.

DeCoster V.A. The emotions of adults with diabetes: a comparison across race. *Soc Work Health Care* 2003;36(4):79–99.

Gans K. Cultural considerations. In: Deen D. & Hark L., eds. *The Complete Guide to Nutrition in Primary Care.* Blackwell Publishing, Malden, MA, 2007.

Gary T.L., Narayan K.M., Gregg E.W., Beckles G.L., Saaddine J.B. Racial/ethnic differences in the healthcare experience (coverage, utilization, and satisfaction) of U.S. adults with diabetes. *Ethn Dis* 2003;13(1):47–54.

Health Disparities Collaboratives. A national effort to improve health outcomes for all medically underserved people with chronic diseases. Diabetes Disease Collaborative. Available at: http://www.healthdisparities.net/hdc/html/home.aspx.

Hunt L.M., Arar N.H., Akana L.L. Herbs, prayer, and insulin. Use of medical and alternative treatments by a group of Mexican-American diabetes patients. *J Fam Pract* 2000;49(3):216–23.

Jezewski M.A., Poss J. Mexican-Americans' explanatory model of type 2 diabetes. *West J Nurs Res* 2002;24(8):840–58.

Oomen J.S., Owen L.J., Suggs L.S. Culture counts: why current treatment models fail Hispanic women with type 2 diabetes. *Diabetes Educ* 1999;25(2):220–5.

Poss J., Jezewski M.A. The role and meaning of susto in Mexican-Americans' explanatory model of type 2 diabetes. *Med Anthropol Q* 2002;16(3):360–77.

Poss J.E., Jezewski M.A., Stuart A.G. Home remedies for type 2 diabetes used by Mexican-Americans in El Paso, Texas. *Clin Nurs Res* 2003;12(4):304–23.

Walsh M.E., Katz M.A., Sechrest L. Unpacking cultural factors in adaptation to type 2 diabetes mellitus. *Med Care* 2002;40(1):I129–39 (suppl).

Weller S.C., Baer R.D., Pachter L.M., et al. Latino beliefs about diabetes. *Diabetes Care* 1999;22(5):722–8.

Wen L.K., Parchman M.L., Shepherd M.D. Family support and diet barriers among older Hispanic adults with type 2 diabetes. *Fam Med* 2004;36(6):423–30.

CASE 4
Maya Mohammed

A 15-year-old Arab American teenager with leukemia

Amal Mohamed Osman Khidir, MD, FAAP,[1] Alexander Chou, MD,[2] and Lyuba Konopasek, MD, FAAP[3]

[1] Weill Cornell Medical College in Qatar, Doha, Qatar
[2] Memorial Sloan-Kettering Cancer Center, New York, NY, USA
[3] Weill Cornell Medical College, New York, NY, USA

Educational Objectives

- Distinguish between religious and cultural traditions of Arab Americans.
- Identify potential sensitivities in communicating and in performing a physical exam while caring for Muslim teens.
- Identify support systems for an Arab/Muslim family with a child who has a serious illness.
- Describe Islamic dietary laws that should be considered in the care of a hospitalized Muslim teen.

TACCT Domains: 2, 3, 4

Case Summary, Questions and Answers

Maya Mohammed is a 15-year-old Arab American teenage girl who comes in with her mother, Mrs. Ali,* because she has not been feeling well. She is scheduled to see the on-call pediatrician, Dr. John Brown. Maya's family immigrated from Jordan 1 year ago. Maya and her

---

Achieving Cultural Competency: A case-based approach to training health professionals,
1st edition. Edited by L Hark, H DeLisser. © 2009 Blackwell Publishing,
ISBN: 9781405180726.

mother are both Muslims and are wearing a hijab, a traditional head covering. At the beginning of the interview, Maya states that she is too tired to talk and Mrs. Ali explains that Maya has lost weight, has had abdominal pain, is tired, and feels achy all the time. After getting more history from the mother, Dr. Brown asks to speak with Maya alone for a few minutes. After Mrs. Ali leaves the room, Dr. Brown asks Maya if she is sexually active and if she could be pregnant. At this point, Maya denies this in an angry tone and states that she wants her mom. When Mrs. Ali returns and asks Maya why she is upset, Maya tells her mother that the doctor is asking if she is pregnant. She explains that she is tired and wants to go home. Mrs. Ali asks Dr. Brown about what happened, and he explains that this is a routine question asked of all female patients with her symptoms. Mrs. Ali tries to soothe Maya by saying, "Maya, he is just doing his job, just be patient." She then turns to the doctor and explains that it is forbidden to have sex out of wedlock in the Muslim religion and even asking the question can be taken as a serious insult.

Dr. Brown acknowledges that this is a difficult question, apologizes, and then gives Maya the choice to be examined alone or with her mother. Maya states that she would like her mother to stay in the room. The mother also states that she would like Maya to be examined by a female physician instead of by Dr. Brown. In fact, the triage nurse had already anticipated this need and had suggested that this may be an issue; however, there are no other physicians in the office today.

*Surnames are different because Arab women usually keep their own family name after marriage.

1   Is it appropriate that Dr. Brown asked about sexual activity and how should he respond to Maya's reaction?

All adolescents should be asked about their sexual history. Because Maya's complaints included abdominal pain and fatigue, it is appropriate to include sexually transmitted diseases and pregnancy in the differential diagnosis. It is important to understand that, although this may be a potentially sensitive area for this Muslim teen, the question needs to be asked if it is medically indicated. It is inappropriate to avoid asking these questions based on assumptions of religious observance or acculturation, as this could lead to health care disparities. The question should be asked with sensitivity and attention to the teen's nonverbal responses. Also, it could be framed as a routine question that is asked of all teenage girls with these complaints. It is also important to reinforce the rules surrounding confidentiality; information that a teen discloses related to sexual activity and illegal substance use must remain confidential unless the teen chooses to disclose it or if the situation is life threatening. One should stay conscious of the fact that, in spite of Maya's reaction and that premarital sexual activity is forbidden in the Muslim community, it is still possible that she may be sexually active.

It is also important to respond to Maya's anger about this question by first acknowledging her emotions. Begin by explaining that this is a routine question asked of all teens with these types of symptoms and apologize if the question was upsetting. Noting her religion, it would be appropriate to apologize in advance for having to ask a question that might otherwise cause offense. Remaining flexible is the key in this situation. Although most adolescents are examined alone, this can be adjusted according to the level of comfort of the patient.

2   What would be the most appropriate response to this request for a female physician?

Although a female doctor would be preferable for the examination of a teen girl, most Muslims will adjust to what is medically necessary. It would be important for the physician to reiterate that he understands her preference, but that there are no female physicians available and the examination is essential and a medical necessity. Although it is important to drape every patient correctly, in this case, conservative draping, exposing only the area being examined at any one time, would be especially important. The physician should explain the examination as it is done and continue to reassure the child during the course of the examination. It should also be specifically stated that the patient or parent should inform the health care providers if any part of the exam is unacceptable to them for any reason. If this is a part of the examination that is medically necessary, then a solution will need to be negotiated.

> *Maya and her mother agree to an exam by Dr. Brown. Maya lies down reluctantly, but by the end of the examination, she seems more comfortable. Her physical examination is significant only for the fact*

that Maya appears tired and pale. Dr. Brown draws a CBC to be run in his office lab. These lab studies reveal anemia (Hgb < 7 mg/dL), thrombocytopenia (platelet count 25,000), and leukocytosis (WBC 50,000) with abnormal lymphocytes. Dr. Brown suspects leukemia and requests to speak with Mrs. Ali alone without Maya. Even though Mrs. Ali's English seems fairly good, Dr. Brown requests an Arabic interpreter using the language link phone to make sure Mrs. Ali understands the urgency of the matter and the need for Maya to go immediately to the Emergency Department (ED). Dr. Brown explains that he is very concerned about these lab findings and this is possibly a very serious illness.

Mrs. Ali does not ask any other questions but asks Dr. Brown to call her husband to explain this to him also. Dr. Brown agrees and takes Mr. Mohammed's telephone number. Mrs. Ali states, "I will go to the ED, insha'Allah."

At this point, Dr. Brown feels that Mrs. Ali understands the need to go immediately to the ED and notifies the ED that they are coming shortly. Dr. Brown gets busy and forgets to call Mr. Mohammed.

Several hours later, the ED attending calls Dr. Brown to report that Maya has not yet arrived. Dr. Brown immediately calls Mrs. Ali at home and apologizes for not calling her husband yet and asks why she has not taken Maya to the ED. Mrs. Ali admits that she has not managed to speak to her husband either and is waiting for him to come home prior to taking Maya to the ED.

Definition of insha'Allah

Insha'Allah means "God willing" or "If it is God's will." It is commonly used by Muslims for any commitment to an event in the future. Some Islamic scholars have stated that it is obligatory for a Muslim to use this phrase when referring to any event in the future.

3   Despite the physician's efforts to ensure that she understood the urgency, why did Mrs. Ali go home rather than to the ED?

In Arab and Muslim cultures, a wife is generally expected to get the permission of her husband for all major decisions, although wives do actively participate in this process. Medical emergencies are exceptions to this rule. Mrs. Ali could respond to the situation in the following ways:

- going to the ED and then contacting her husband,
- making every effort to contact her husband and then going to the ED, or
- going home and waiting for her husband to discuss the matter and get permission.

Mrs. Ali's response depends on how much she understands the urgency and time factor as well as how she and her husband deal with these types of decisions. She might have been more likely to go to the ED immediately, even without reaching her husband, if Dr. Brown had been more explicit and explained to her that her daughter may have cancer.

The degree of male dominance is mainly a cultural one and may differ according to the person's country of origin and cultural practice. Consequently, the physician needs to be sensitive to this as a potential issue and should clarify how each individual family makes decisions. It is likely that this case would have gone more smoothly if Dr. Brown had called Mr. Mohammed when Mrs. Ali was still in the office, so that a plan could be negotiated with both parents at the same time.

> *Dr. Brown explains the urgency of the problem again, stating that it is very important that Maya go to the ED as soon as possible because he is concerned that she is very ill. Dr. Brown then arranges a call with Mr. Mohammed with an interpreter. Shortly afterwards, Mrs. Ali and Mr. Mohammed register Maya to the ED. Mr. Mohammed requests that his daughter be examined only by female doctors and nurses and also requests that they respect their religious customs, which require that women remain covered in front of men. The ED doctor explains that they will do their best to honor his requests.*

4   How should the physician and staff respond to the father's requests?

Although both of Maya's parents may be Arab and Muslim, they may differ in their cultural practice or religious belief. Therefore, it is important to determine each parent's individual perspective. In this case, both parents agree that any male, regardless of his title, should knock on the door and ask for permission to enter because Maya will need to have time to put on her hijab. The physicians can reassure the family that they will be mindful of this concern. This is mainly a religious issue because, in the Muslim faith, women are considered tempting for men. The whole body is considered potentially provocative. According to the Qur'an ("holy book"), a woman is to cover her entire body and hair, and the only people who may see a woman without her hijab are her husband, brothers, father, grandfather, uncle, father-in-law, and the woman's children and grandchildren. Young boys can see a woman without her hijab until they can discriminate between men and women. Also, according to the Muslim faith, men and women should always cover the region of the body from the umbilicus to the knee.

Additional tests are performed. A few hours later, Maya's lab tests confirm the initial diagnosis of leukemia. Mr. Mohammed and Mrs. Ali are told by the oncologist through an interpreter in a private setting that their daughter has "leukemia, a type of cancer." Upon hearing this news, Mr. Mohammed takes his head in his hands and Mrs. Ali begins to cry. The oncologist gives the family some time to absorb the news and then explains that Maya needs to be admitted for further testing and to start chemotherapy, the recommended treatment. Mr. Mohammed, with eyes full of tears, agrees to the hospitalization but states that he does not want his daughter to receive chemotherapy at this time. He asks if he can take a few days to think about it and then asks how much time he has so as not to jeopardize her health. He also insists that his daughter not be told of the diagnosis until he has time to prepare her. Mrs. Ali, who has been crying quietly through all of this, now begins to ask clarifying questions about the side effects of the chemotherapy. She does not explicitly state her opinion about the initiation of chemotherapy.

Mr. Mohammad and Mrs. Ali come back into Maya's room, and she asks them what is wrong. Mrs. Ali replies, "Don't worry; the doctors need to do more and they need to keep you in the hospital."

---

5 How could the team resolve this conflict and begin to form a therapeutic alliance with the parents?

The first step would be to elicit the father's perspective and try to understand his reasons for not wanting to tell Maya about her diagnosis, as well as his need for a few days to decide about chemotherapy. It is unlikely that either issue is related to practice of Islam. Mr. Mohammed's statement that he does not want to disclose the diagnosis to Maya is likely a desire, based on his culture, to protect his daughter from bad news. Whereas breaking the news to Maya is something that can continue to be discussed, the issue of chemotherapy needs to be resolved quickly. One potential reason for Mr. Mohammed's request for more time may be to discuss the situation with other family members particularly if they are physicians. The extended family is extremely important in Arab culture. Mr. Mohammed will likely want to consult with family members, particularly if they are physicians, who may live abroad. Anticipating this, it is important for the physician to clarify that, if there are any family members who will call him, he has permission to talk to them, and to establish the rules of confidentiality. Family members may call because they are concerned about the patient, but also because the father consulted with them. It is useful to identify one or two people, in addition to the mother and father, who would be the main family contacts. It is also important to anticipate that Maya will have many visitors and clarify hospital regulations and plans up front.

6 Should Mrs. Ali's opinion about chemotherapy be asked directly in front of her husband?

Asking Mrs. Ali directly has the potential to make the situation more difficult. Even if she agrees that Maya should receive immediate chemotherapy, it is likely that she will not want to contradict her husband explicitly in public for both cultural and religious reasons. However, it is certainly important to elicit her opinion. Also, she may involve other family members, especially more senior ones, who may share her opinion and influence her husband.

In forming a therapeutic alliance with Mr. Mohammed and Mrs. Ali, it is important to first elicit an explanatory model of leukemia and cancer in general, as described in Appendix 2. This is an important early step in shared and informed decision making. Table 4.1 shows a model to establish a shared and informed decision-making process.

> *After further discussion with Mr. Mohammed about his understanding of leukemia, the physician learns that Mr. Mohammed views the diagnosis of leukemia as a death sentence, based on his experience with a second cousin who died of this illness. He therefore wants to consult with his brother, who is a physician in the U.S. The team explains that, although leukemia is a very serious illness, chemotherapy can be curative,*

> and it will be important to admit Maya for further testing to find out what kind of leukemia she has. Furthermore, they offer to speak with Mr. Mohammad's brother. A day later, Mr. Mohammed and Mrs. Ali agree to the chemotherapy, stating that they want to be very involved in all of the decisions of Maya's treatment. However, Mr. Mohammed re-iterates that he does not want anyone to tell Maya about her diagnosis yet. The team commits to discussing all aspects of care with him.
>
> By the end of the week, Mr. Mohammed, in consultation with Mrs. Ali and the rest of the family, decides that Maya should be told of her diagnosis. He states that their imam, the person who leads prayers in their mosque, and one of the family elders will do this with him. In general, both religious and cultural beliefs are to have one or two people with wisdom and faith when breaking bad news.

7   Are there any issues related to Maya's care in the hospital that should be considered in the context of this family's culture and their belief in Islam?

Aside from the issues regarding privacy that have been discussed, the health care team should consider rules surrounding diet and hygiene. Islamic dietary laws specify which foods are halal (lawful) and which foods are haram (taboo). Pork is forbidden, and gelatin products, many of which are made from pork, may also be haram. In addition, meat should be slaughtered according to specific rules to be considered halal. Thus, depending on the degree of religious observance, patients may find it easiest to choose a vegetarian diet in

Table 4.1 Towle's competencies for informed shared decision making

---

- Build a partnership with the patient/family.
- Consider and reestablish patient's preferences for role in decision making.
- Elicit patient's and family's views on diagnosis and management and respond to patient's ideas, views, and concerns.
- Identify choices and evaluate research evidence.
- Present evidence, keeping in mind how much the patient wants to know and how much they want to participate in decision making; help patient reflect on effects on lifestyle.
- Make or negotiate a decision and check that it is acceptable to all.
- Agree on an action plan and complete arrangements for follow-up.

Source: Adapted from Towle A., Godophin W. Framework for teaching and learning informed shared decision making. *Br Med J* 1999;319:766–71.

the hospital and have it supplemented by food brought in by family members.

Cleanliness is considered extremely important in the practice of Islam, and there are specific rules related to hygiene that must be considered. Blood on the body or on clothing should be cleaned up as soon as possible. However, if it relates directly to the illness, such as blood at the dressing site, it is not necessary to change it. Ritual washing with water, wudu (partial ablution), is necessary prior to any of the five daily prayers. Ghusl (full ablution) is a requirement for continuing prayer after menstruation. Wudu can be done in the bed using a wash basin. Ghusl involves a certain sequence of washing and generally needs to be done in a shower or bath, but could be accomplished in bed. If there is a medical reason, a patient can do wudu and not do ghusl to prepare for praying. Again, an imam can help a family with these types of issues. Finally, in the context of culture, visiting the sick by family, friends, and acquaintances is the norm. Plans for this, especially when the patient is immunocompromised, should be discussed in advance.

Finally, it should be considered that a family's practice and degree of observance may actually change during the course of care. Errihani's study of the impact of a cancer diagnosis on Moroccan patients of the Muslim faith demonstrated that many nonobservant Muslims became more observant after the cancer diagnosis.

> *Maya receives chemotherapy treatments for 2 years. During her course of chemotherapy, the religious holiday Ramadan begins. During this 1-month spiritual cleansing period, Muslims fast during the day and eat only after sundown until just before sunrise. During the daytime, they cannot eat, drink water, or smoke. Maya states that she wants to fast. The team is concerned because she will not be able to consume adequate calories, protein, or fluids to meet her requirements.*

8 What are the rules surrounding Ramadan, children, and the sick? What is the best way to support Maya in her spiritual beliefs while attending to her health care needs?

In Islam, any child who has reached puberty is required to observe Ramadan; however, many parents encourage younger children to practice by fasting for at least part of the day. In this case, the imam might be consulted for clarification. Mr. Mohammed and Mrs. Ali

will be observing Ramadan. As their main meal will be around sun-
set, this may affect their visiting times and the schedule of team
meetings. The sick, elderly, pregnant, and nursing women are ex-
cused from fasting at Ramadan. It will be important to clarify the
parents' opinion on whether or not they agree with Maya's plan to
fast. Again, either way, an imam could be brought in to help resolve
this issue. Even if Maya does not fast during Ramadan, she can pray.
She does not need to go anywhere or even sit up to pray; she can
pray lying down if needed. In Islam, it is said that a sick person can
even pray by using their finger, and if they cannot move their finger,
they can use their eyes.

> *Four months after Maya completes chemotherapy, she relapses and
> fails additional treatment. There are no additional options for curative
> chemotherapy, and a plan for palliative care is discussed with Maya and
> her family.*

9   How can Maya's terminal illness be communicated to her and her family in a culturally appropriate manner?

Given that Maya is not yet 18 years old, it would be important to
first speak with her parents. In Islam, a central teaching is that only
Allah knows when it is time for a person to die. Thus, this conversation should begin with the statement that no person knows when,
where, or how someone will die. This type of statement may give
Maya's parents the trust that their health care provider is sensitive to
their beliefs. If there is a question about prognosis, the physician can
phrase it as, "In my experience with others, it may occur . . . " Gatrad
suggests "show(ing) guarded confidence, yet discuss(ing) the real
possibility of worse to come, sometimes suddenly and catastrophi-
cally." Potentially, involving a Muslim physician in these discussions
may help because they will be perceived as understanding and sharing the Muslim family's worldview, as well as being able to bring
their medical expertise. As Gatrad states, the Muslim physician can
assert the primacy of the child's interests and discuss difficult decisions in the context of the teachings of Islam. The issue of having
Maya and/or Maya's mother involved in end-of-life conversations is
more cultural than religious. Men sometimes want to be protective
or dominant and do not want children or women to get involved

in decision making. This may be related to the perception that men have a higher tolerance for pain and agony.

10 Are there issues related to the family's religious beliefs that may impact on a palliative care plan?

In Islam, pain is managed both with medication and through spiritual means. Overall, Islam encourages people to increase their patience, tolerance, and acceptance of unfavorable situations. Such situations are accepted as either a test or a punishment. Each person will have his/her own interpretation of whether it is a test or a punishment. If it is a test, Muslims are encouraged to be patient. If it is a punishment, Muslims are encouraged to continue asking Allah ("God") for forgiveness and cure. In Maya's situation, the imam will be helpful in giving support and prayer. The perspectives of the parents and/or Maya may contribute to decisions about pain management. Finally, Muslims use the Qur'an for both spiritual and physical treatment, either on their own or with the assistance of an imam.

Finally, a conversation about plans for "Do Not Resuscitate" orders needs to be conducted with special sensitivity, as this aspect of care is a complex issue in Muslim communities. Again, it will be helpful to involve an imam and a Muslim physician in this conversation.

11 How might the team provide culturally relevant and appropriate comfort and support to this patient and her family?

At the end of life, some Muslims prefer to be released to go home or even travel to Mecca in Saudi Arabia. When Maya is in the hospital, she will pray and read the Qur'an in her room. Facilitating visits by the imam or a religious person to support her and her family will also be extremely helpful. Furthermore, negotiating a plan for other visitors is essential. Muslims are encouraged to support and visit the ill. Sometimes Muslims just go and visit a sick Muslim in the hospital even if they do not have a relationship with the patient. With some patience and preparedness, the staff can support the family without violating the visitation, isolation, or HIPAA policies. Visitors can be with the family in the waiting room if the patient is in isolation or within a limited visitation status.

References: Case 4

da Costa D.E., Ghazal H., Khusaiby S.A., Gatrad A.R. Do Not Resuscitate orders and ethical decisions in a neonatal intensive care unit in a Muslim community. *Arch Dis Child Fetal Neonatal Ed* 2002;86:115–9.

Errihani H., Mrabti H., Boutayeb S., et al. Impact of cancer on Moslem patients in Morocco. *Psycho-Oncology* 2008;17(1):98–100.

Gatrad A.R., Sheikh A. Medical ethics and Islam: principles and practice *Arch Dis Child* 2001;84:72–5.

Gatrad A.R., Sheikh A. Palliative care for Muslims and issues before death *Intern J Palliative Nursing* 2002;8:526–31.

McKean E. (ed). *New Oxford American Dictionary*, 2nd ed. New York, Oxford University Press, 2005.

Oxford-American Dictionary for definition of "imam." Towle A., Godophin W. Framework for teaching and learning shared decision making. *Br Med J* 1999;319:766–71.

CASE 5

Jon Le

A 48-year-old Korean man with cerebral hemorrhage

Scott Kasner, MD, and Horace DeLisser, MD
University of Pennsylvania School of Medicine, Philadelphia, PA, USA

Educational Objectives

- Take into account that ethnic and cultural heritage may affect medical decision making with regard to when and how a patient seeks treatment.
- Describe how to approach patients who desire to use complementary and alternative medicine.
- Know that differences exist within cultures that Westerners may view as a homogeneous group.

TACCT Domains: 1, 3, 4, 6

Case Summary, Questions and Answers

Mr. Le is a 48-year-old Korean American engineer who has been a U.S. resident for the last 20 years. His wife died 10 years ago and he has one daughter, age 26. He develops a sudden headache and left-sided facial drooping with left arm weakness while having lunch with his daughter. His daughter insists (to the point of tears) that he should go immediately to the hospital, but he first seeks treatment from a practitioner of Chinese medicine for "moxibustion" heat therapy.

Achieving Cultural Competency: A case-based approach to training health professionals,
1st edition. Edited by L Hark, H DeLisser. © 2009 Blackwell Publishing,
ISBN: 9781405180726.

Moxibustion

Moxibustion, or moxa, is one the major healing modalities of traditional Chinese medicine. It involves the application of heat generated by the burning of mugwort, a small, spongy herb, at targeted acupuncture points. As with all aspects of traditional Chinese medicine, the goal of this therapy is to strengthen the blood, stimulate the flow of *qi* (also known as *chi*, the energy of life) and support overall health. It has been widely used to treat a variety of diseases and conditions, including breech birth, Hashimoto disease, rheumatoid arthritis, menstrual cramps, and musculoskeletal pain or inflammation.

There are two types of Moxibustion: direct and indirect. In direct moxibustion, a small cone-shaped amount of the ground-up mugwort is placed over an acupuncture point and burned on the skin. The ignited herb may be allowed to burn itself out, resulting in blistering and localized scarring after healing (scarring moxibustion), or it may be extinguished or removed before injury to the skin (nonscarring moxibustion). In indirect moxibustion, the mugwort does not have direct contact with the skin. Instead, a burning, cigar-size stick of the mugwort is held close to the area being treated until the skin turns red, or an acupuncture needle is placed into an acupoint and the free end of the needle is wrapped with the herb and ignited. Indirect moxibustion is more popular because of the lower risk of pain or burning.

1 How does this patient's heritage and culture affect his decision-making process with regard to his current medical condition?

Acculturation describes the process by which the values, attitudes, and behaviors of individuals from one culture are changed over time as a result of contact with a new and different culture. Regardless of how it is conceptualized, acculturation occurs across multiple domains (e.g. attitudes, values, self-identification, language/communication, customs, etc.), the pace and pattern of which is dependent on many factors, including age, gender, length of time in the U.S., literacy level, language proficiency, and the nature of contacts with the host culture. Although Mr. Le has been in the U.S. for 20 years and is employed as an engineer, it should not be assumed that he has completely assimilated into American and/or Western culture. Traditional Eastern concepts of health and healing might still be significant and relevant to him. Given the large number of factors that influence rates of integration or assimilation into the dominant culture, it is not surprising that differing patterns of acculturation among family members can occur, leading to intergenerational conflict between parents and children.

The impact of acculturation on health-related outcomes is complex. Low levels of acculturation may compromise access to, or utilization of, effective Western treatments, potentially leading to health-related disparities (as in Mr. Le's case). In addition, individuals who have experienced a high level of acculturation, particularly with respect to adopting a Western diet and sedentary lifestyle, typically have poorer outcomes. Studies of first- and second-generation U.S. immigrants have demonstrated that acculturation is associated with increased morbidity and mortality from a number of chronic degenerative diseases.

Assimilation and Acculturation

There are a number of assimilation models; two such models have been proposed to describe the process of acculturation. The first is a unidimensional, zero-sum scheme model in which individuals adopting host-culture values and behaviors simultaneously discard or relinquish the corresponding attributes from their native culture. This model of acculturation is conceived as a single continuum of change, in which some will quickly and strongly adopt the cultural values, practices, and behaviors of their new country, readily relinquishing their original culture (assimilationists), whereas a number of them (at least initially) will choose to hold tightly to the culture of their origin, despite daily contact with the host culture (separationists). Between these low and high levels of acculturation are others who, to varying degrees, will try to maintain their culture of origin while selectively embracing elements of the host culture (integrationist).

In contrast to this unidimensional model of acculturation, a second model has more recently emerged that conceptualizes acculturation as more often a *bidimensional* process in which there is high adherence to both the native and the host culture and that both the old and new cultures for the individual may change independently of each other, so changes in one may not be associated with reciprocal changes in the other. For example, the Korean immigrant becoming "less Korean" over time does not necessarily mean that s/he has become more American; or that, as the immigrant becomes "more American," s/he may still maintain a high identity to Korean culture. Because self-defined identity is not the same thing as behavior, many immigrants identify as being American and maintain family traditions and values. Evidence of this comes from studies of the use of traditional health care among Korean Americans, which have shown that the most educated and acculturated Korean immigrants are actually more likely to seek traditional healing than those less acculturated and of lower socioeconomic status. In fact, the majority of users of alternative medical care in the U.S. are white, college-educated individuals.

Several hours later, when moxibustion therapy did not improve his symptoms, Mr. Le agrees to go to the Emergency Department (ED). As the ED resident evaluates Mr. Le, he notices first- and second-degree burns on his arms and legs. The physician wants to treat the burns, but Mr. Le is hesitant, fearing that this will counteract the beneficial effects of the moxibustion treatment.

2   How should the physician approach Mr. Le about his use of alternative medicine?

Complementary and alternative medicine (CAM) encompasses a diverse group of treatments currently not included in conventional medicine. When combined with conventional interventions, these approaches are referred to as "complementary medicine," whereas "alternative medicine" describes modalities that are used in place of conventional medicine. Various personal, societal, and cultural factors may lead a patient to seek CAM. The National Center for Complementary and Alternative Medicine has separated CAM into five domains:

- *Whole medical systems* (e.g. homeopathy, naturopathy, traditional Chinese medicine, and Ayurveda).
- *Mind–body medicine* approaches that aim to enhance the mind's capacity to affect the body (e.g. mindfulness meditation).
- *Biologically based practices* (e.g. herbal or dietary supplements and products).
- *Manipulative and body-based practices* (e.g. chiropractic medicine, osteopathic manipulation).
- *Energy medicine,* in which purported energy fields around an individual are manipulated (e.g. acupuncture, moxibustion).

The use of these modalities, particularly when they involve the use of alternative medical systems, may be part of a strong cultural identity. When the physician learns about the patient's CAM usage, if he or she responds with visible shock, amazement, or disgust, it is likely to alienate Mr. Le. Although there is obvious concern about injury or harm from Mr. Le's use of CAM, the physician needs to initiate a nonjudgmental, respectful conversation with the patient. In the end, the goal is to develop a relationship in which the patient is willing to be candid with the physician about all aspects of his/her health. The patient and his health care providers will need to try to develop a consensus regarding a realistic and achievable treatment plan. Fundamentally there is no interaction between antihypertensive therapy and moxibustion, so they can be used simultaneously. However, the key to prevention of recurrent cerebral hemorrhage is aggressive blood pressure control. It is possible that other traditional Chinese medicines could interact with his prescribed antihypertensive agents, so again, a relationship with open and ongoing communication is critical to ensure optimal care.

> *Mr. Le overhears the resident explaining his case to the attending physician outside his door. On more than one occasion during the conversation, the resident refers to Mr. Le as a Chinese man, even though he is Korean. When the attending enters the room, Mr. Le is noticeably angry and hostile and therefore not forthcoming with any answers to the attending's questions.*

3   Why is Mr. Le angry and how could this have been avoided?

Individuals who trace their origins to the Far East, Southeast Asia, or the Indian subcontinent now comprise 5% of the U.S. population (or nearly 15 million people). This "Asian" population, like all ethnic groups, is not homogenous, but instead constitutes several diverse and culturally distinct subgroups, each with specific identities. Some Asian groups, such as the Japanese and Chinese, have had histories in the U.S. that go back several generations, whereas others, such as Koreans, Vietnamese, Hmong, Cambodians, and other South Asians, are more recent arrivals. Suffice it to say, respecting the diversity of patients of Asian ancestry by asking and identifying based on the patient's preference is essential. Historically, and especially for

first-generation immigrants, lingering tensions from previous conflicts, such as that between the Japanese and Chinese or Koreans
during World War II, may create added sensitivity about being ethnically misidentified. Where there is uncertainty, simply ask the following questions to avoid an unintended insult:
- *Where were you born?*
- *Where does your family, generations back, come from?*
- *What ethnic identity best describes you?*

> Mr. Le undergoes a CT scan that reveals a small intracerebral hemor-
> rhage. He is subsequently admitted to the neurology service and found
> to have significant hypertension, which ultimately requires three medi-
> cations to control. Mr. Le is reluctant to take them but eventually agrees.
> Prior to his discharge, he asks his daughter to call his traditional Chinese
> medicine (TCM) practitioner to prepare herbal remedy, as he does not
> plan to take any of the blood pressure medications he is receiving in the
> hospital after he is discharged. His daughter informs the physician of his
> intentions.

4   How should the physician approach Mr. Le about his plan to work with a TCM physician?

In responding to Mr. Le, the central tasks are to first obtain a real
understanding of the patient's worldview with respect to health and
healing and then use that information as a basis for dialogue and negotiation with the patient. For facilitating these kinds of potentially
challenging cross-cultural conversations, Berlin and colleagues have
offered an approach that goes by the acronym LEARN:
- **L**isten with sympathy and understanding to the patient's perception of the problem.
- **E**xplain your (medical) perceptions and understandings of the
  problem.
- **A**cknowledge and discuss differences and similarities.
- **R**ecommend treatment.
- **N**egotiate agreement.

Questions that can be used to initiate the process of "LEARNing"
and to begin to explore the meaning and significance of disease to
the patient include:
- *What do you think has caused your problem?*
- *What do you think your sickness does to you?*
- *Why do you think it started when it did?*

- *How severe is your sickness?*
- *What kind of treatment do you think you should receive?*

References: Case 5

Abe-Kim J., Okazaki S., Goto S.G. Unidimensional versus multidimensional approaches to the assessment of acculturation for Asian American populations. *Cultur Divers Ethnic Minor Psychol* 2001;7:232–46.

Berlin E.A., Fowkes W.C. Teaching framework for cross-cultural care: application in family practice. *West J Med* 1983;6:934–8.

Broderick J., Connolly S., Feldmann E., et al. Guidelines for the management of spontaneous intracerebral hemorrhage in adults: 2007 update: a guideline from the American Heart Association/American Stroke Association, Stroke Council, High Blood Pressure Research Council, and the quality of care and outcomes in research interdisciplinary working group. *Stroke* 2007;38:2001–23.

Carrillo J.E., Green A.R., Betancourt J.R. Cross-cultural primary care: a patient-based approach. *Ann Intern Med* 1999;130(10):829–34.

Choi G.S., Han J.B., Park J.H., et al. Effects of moxibustion to zusanli (ST36) on alteration of natural killer cell activity in rats. *Am J Chin Med* 2004;32:303–12.

Chung R.H. Gender, ethnicity, and acculturation in intergenerational conflict of Asian American college students. *Cultur Divers Ethnic Minor Psychol* 2001;7:376–86.

Cirigliano M. Advising patients about herbal therapies. *JAMA* 1998;280:1565–6.

Frisbie W.P., Cho Y., Hummer R.A. Immigration and the health of Asian and Pacific Islander adults in the United States. *Am J Epidemiol* 2001;153:372–80.

Kanakura Y., Kometani K., Nagata T., et al. Moxibustion treatment of breech presentation. *Am J Chin Med* 2001;29:37–45.

Kim B.S., Yang P.H., Atkinson D.R., Wolfe M.M., Hong S. Cultural value similarities and differences among Asian American ethnic groups. *Cultur Divers Ethnic Minor Psychol* 2001;7:343–61.

Kim J., Chan M.M. Acculturation and dietary habits of Korean Americans. *Br J Nutr* 2004;91:469–78.

Kim J., Chan M.M. Factors influencing preferences for alternative medicine by Korean Americans. *Am J Chin Med* 2004;32:321–9.

Kleinman A., Eisenberg L., Good B. Culture, illness, and care: clinical lessons from anthropological and cross-cultural research. *Ann Intern Med* 1978;88:251–88.

Lee R.M., Falbo T., Doh H.S., Park SY. The Korean diasporic experience: measuring ethnic identity in the United States and China. *Cultur Divers Ethnic Minor Psychol* 2001;7:207–16.

Leong F.T. The role of acculturation in the career adjustment of Asian American workers: a test of Leong and Chou's (1994) formulations. *Cultur Divers Ethnic Minor Psychol* 2001;7:262–73.

Liem R., Lim B.A., Liem J.H. Acculturation and emotion among Asian Americans. *Cultur Divers Ethnic Minor Psychol* 2000;6(1):13–31.

National Center for Complementary and Alternative Medicine. What is CAM? Available at: http://www.nccam.nih.gov.

Unger J.B., Reynolds K., Shakib S., Spruijt-Metz D., Sun P., Johnson C.A. Acculturation, physical activity, and fast-food consumption among Asian-American and Hispanic adolescents. *J Community Health* 2004;29:467–81.

U.S. Census Bureau. Annual Estimates of the Population by Sex, Race, and Hispanic or Latino Origin for the United States: April 1, 2000 to July 1, 2006 (NC-EST2006-03). Available at: http://www.census.gov.

CASE 6

Nadia Rosenberg

A 53-year-old Russian woman with drug-resistant tuberculosis

Elena N. Atochina-Vasserman, MD, PhD, and Helen Abramova, MD
University of Pennsylvania School of Medicine, Philadelphia, PA, USA

Educational Objectives

- Review the importance of obtaining an interpreter to facilitate effective communication and good care.
- Examine some the challenges that arise when using a medical interpreter.
- Identify that previous health-related experiences of individuals from other societies may represent a barrier to their care in America.
- Propose that unappreciated cultural beliefs or practices can result in misunderstandings that interfere with patient–physician dialogue.

TACCT Domains: 4, 5

Case Summary, Questions and Answers

Nadia Rosenberg is a 53-year-old Russian woman who immigrated to the United States with her husband and two teenage children 3 years ago. She works 6 days a week as a housekeeper (although she was previously

Achieving Cultural Competency: A case-based approach to training health professionals,
1st edition. Edited by L Hark, H DeLisser. © 2009 Blackwell Publishing,
ISBN: 9781405180726.

a University history professor in Russia). Her husband is employed as a seasonal construction worker. As a result of her income, they are able to afford some limited medical insurance. Her health has been good, and she has not seen a physician in the United States since she immigrated. However, over the last several weeks, she has begun experiencing a persistent cough. She has never smoked and initially attributed the cough to her exposure to cleaning solutions but became alarmed when she began to see streaks of blood in her sputum. She is not experiencing any fever, chills, or weight loss and otherwise feels fine. Because she is coughing up blood, she goes to the Emergency Department (ED) of a local hospital, where the waiting area is overflowing with patients waiting to be seen. After being evaluated by the triage nurse, she is instructed to remain in the waiting area until she is called to be seen. However, she approaches the registration desk every 15 to 20 minutes to ask when she will see a physician. Each time, she is instructed to return to her seat and is told, "We will call you when the doctor is ready." After 3 hours, she leaves without being seen.

1   Given that the waits for nonemergent care in many EDs are usually long, why was Mrs. Rosenberg so impatient and decided to leave?

It goes without saying that, for most people in the United States, regardless of their background, long waits in an ED (whether real or perceived) before being evaluated would be a source of frustration. However, this frustration may be more pronounced given Mrs. Rosenberg's recent immigration from Russia.

Health care in other societies is organized very differently from the American system, and the experience of illness and its treatment in this country may be very alien to immigrants. Thus, for Mrs. Rosenberg, her impatience and frustration at the "long wait," and her subsequent departure without being seen, reflect the fact that, in Russia, the ED principally provides urgent and emergent care and very little primary care. As a result, patients are typically seen very promptly and rarely have to wait to be evaluated, particularly if they are coughing up blood. Furthermore, as Russian doctors routinely make house calls, she thought that if she left she would be able to easily arrange for a doctor to come to her home for a house call. This provides a small illustration of how a past cultural experience could potentially result in an ethnically based, health-related disparity.

> As her English-language skills are very limited, the next day Mrs. Rosenberg asks an English-speaking Russian neighbor to assist her in obtaining an appointment with a lung physician. With the help of the neighbor, she is able to arrange for a visit with a pulmonologist the following week. Not knowing who else to ask, she has the neighbor accompany her to the pulmonologist to serve as an interpreter. As Mrs. Rosenberg waits to be seen, she is particularly fearful of a diagnosis of lung cancer.

2   What issues might result for the patient and the physician when using a neighbor or family member as an interpreter?

Patients with limited English proficiency may bring a friend or family member to their visit with the doctor to serve as an interpreter. In using this type of untrained individual, an accurate interpretation may not always be conveyed to the patient due to the friend's or family member's own limitation with English, lack of medical sophistication and experience, and/or inadequate communication skills. Furthermore, cultural factors may also intrude and distort the process. In Russia, for example, there is a culturally driven mandate to not fully inform patients (as understood in Western terms) of the nature and extent of their diagnosis regarding a terminal illness. Thus, the diagnosis of a metastatic cancer may be conveyed by the Russian interpreter to her Russian friend in a way that does not indicate the advanced nature of the malignancy. That is "опухоль" (a benign, or operable tumor) may be used instead of "РАК" (an incurable cancer). Knowing that patients in Russia may not be informed of the diagnosis of a terminal cancer, the Russian immigrant who is particularly concerned about a cancer may fear that her Russian companion who she brought (or even the physician) will not be completely forthcoming about a cancer diagnosis.

Given the above, trained/professional interpreters or telephone interpreter services are preferred to interpretation provided by ad hoc family members, friends, or available, untrained medical or nonmedical staff. There are, however, some potential limitations should be noted. First, it is important to acknowledge the challenges faced by a trained interpreter in faithfully acting as a neutral, two-way, conduit of information and behavior. Second, the language barrier and the presence of an interpreter inevitably tends to stifle some of the purely social and spontaneous interactions, or "small talk," that could and does occur between patients and physicians who communicate directly with each other in the same language. For groups where this kind of interaction is important, its absence may diminish some of their satisfaction with the physician encounter. Aranguri and coworkers also suggest that the lack of social discourse limits the physician's ability to diagnose for him or herself any psychosocial disorders or compliance/adherence issues related to the social situation of interpreted patients.

Mrs. Rosenberg is seen by a pulmonologist, Dr. Ruth Davies. After the visit, a sputum sample is obtained for acid-fast bacillus (AFB) staining and culture, and a chest x-ray is performed. The chest x-ray reveals an upper lobe infiltrate, raising the question of pulmonary tuberculosis (TB). Although the initial AFB stains were negative, 3 weeks later the cultures confirm the presence of a multidrug-resistant (MDR) strain of tuberculosis. Upon receiving these results, Dr. Davies calls Mrs. Rosenberg on the telephone and explains that she needs immediate treatment and that she should come back to the office the next day to discuss this further. Mrs. Rosenberg says, "okay" to all of Dr. Davies' statements and concludes the call with, "I understand." However, Mrs. Rosenberg did not keep her scheduled appointment the next day. Dr. Davies calls her home multiple times, but is unable to reach her. She leaves several messages on Mrs. Rosenberg's answering machine urging her to make an appointment as soon as possible, but Mrs. Rosenberg fails to do so.

---

3 Why would Mrs. Rosenberg say "okay" and "I understand" but fail to follow-up for further evaluation?

A number of patient-related factors may influence the level of patient adherence to prescribed medications, physician instructions, recommended treatments, or health-promotion activities. These include language barriers, life responsibilities, familial commitments, employment obligations, the level of financial resources, and the quality of health insurance, as well as the psychological and emotional distractions resulting from these factors. Also important are folk or cultural beliefs and the patient's understanding of his/her disease or illness. In addition, actions on the part of the physician may contribute to poor patient adherence. These include failing to establish a trusting patient–physician relationship, prescribing complex treatments, and providing inadequate follow-up or poor instructions.

When Mrs. Rosenberg eventually does come for her visit, Dr. Davies learns that her reasons for not returning promptly were multiple. So, she in fact had not really understood the urgency of what Dr. Davies had said because of her limited English proficiency. When she had tried to call the doctor's office (several times) to make an appointment, she was unable to navigate the phone system to speak to one of the office staff. And in the last week she had completely ignored Dr. Davies' messages and had not tried to get help because she really could not afford to be absent from work. Finally, she admits that, in the back of her mind, she was fearful that she has cancer and was dreading to come to the doctor for the potentially bad news.

Epidemiology of Tuberculosis

The introduction of antituberculosis medications in the late 1940s was followed by a steady decline in the incidence of TB in the United States. However, beginning in the mid-1980s, there was a resurgence in the number of reported cases due to several factors, including: (i) the deterioration of the TB public health infrastructure; (ii) the HIV/AIDS epidemic; (iii) immigration of persons from countries where TB was common; (iv) transmission of TB in congregate settings (e.g. prisons and long-term care and nursing facilities); and (v) emergence of MDR TB. With aggressive public health efforts there have been dramatic decreases in the rates of new TB infections, such that in 2006, 13,767 tuberculosis cases (4.6 cases per 100,000 population) were reported, the lowest recorded since national reporting began in 1953. Racial and ethnic minorities in the United States are disproportionately affected by TB, with 80% of all reported TB cases occurring in racial and ethnic minorities. Much of the increased risk of TB in minorities has been linked to lower socioeconomic status and the effects of crowding.

> *Although the initial AFB stains were negative, 3 weeks later the cultures confirm the presence of a MDR strain of tuberculosis. After several additional failed attempts to schedule an office visit, Dr. Davies decides to call Mrs. Rosenberg's neighbor on the telephone because she was listed as the emergency contact in her chart from the initial visit. Dr. Davies explains the urgency of the matter to the neighbor without disclosing her diagnosis. Through the intervention of the neighbor, Mrs. Rosenberg finally comes back to see Dr. Davies 1 week later, and the office arranges for a trained Russian interpreter to be present for the visit.*

Mrs. Rosenberg answers the question, "What is your understanding of tuberculosis?" *"This is a lung disease that makes people cough up blood; it is highly contagious; and in Russia, you have to live in a special hospital away from your family for many months. Is that what is going to happen to me?"* And, "What do you fear the most?" *"I am worried that I may have infected my husband and children."* This information pertains to a past or current cultural experience that can be used to facilitate the physician–patient relationship and promote patient adherence. In this regard, cancer is a common fear among Russians, and thus, many physicians who care for immigrant patients, such as Mrs. Rosenberg, from the former Soviet Union will begin these kinds of conversations by saying, "You do not have cancer."

Tuberculosis in Russia

After years of gradual decline, the incidence of TB in Russia doubled during the 1990s, although TB incidence rates have stabilized over the last 5 years. Currently, the incidence rates for TB in Russia are 115 new cases per 100,000 people, placing Russia 12th among the 22 countries with high burdens of TB (*WHO Global TB Report 2006*). These numbers reflect the deterioration of the Russian health care system since the collapse of the Soviet Union in the early 1990s. This breakup facilitated the spread of infectious diseases, including TB and MDR TB in many former Soviet Republics.

> *According to the regulations of the City Health Department, Mrs. Rosenberg will have to report three times per week to the Health Department downtown to receive directly observed treatment (DOT) for her tuberculosis. This means a health care worker or another designated person*

observes Mrs. Rosenberg swallow each dose of her medication. When informed of this by Dr. Davies, she becomes very upset and expresses to the interpreter that she does not understand why she needs to take her medication under supervision as if she were a child. "I am an adult." In frustration, Dr. Davies says, "It appears you don't want to get better."

4   Why might Mrs. Rosenberg be so resistant to DOT for her tuberculosis?

Although DOT for tuberculosis is deemed to be the appropriate public health response to the rise in the incidence of tuberculosis, its impact on individual patients and the disruption it might cause in their lives could be significant. Certainly making the effort to ensure that the patient understands the diagnosis and the importance of treatment is a necessary first step in acquiring patient adherence to this therapy. Equally, if not more important, however, is the need to fully understand how DOT will impact the patient's life. This will allow the physician to address and respond to any current issues and anticipate and/or plan for future problems.

Upon further questioning, Mrs. Rosenberg reveals that she does not have a car and will need to take public transportation to and from the public health clinic. This requires two buses and 1.5 hours each way, as well as the cost of the bus fare. With some frustration she notes that, in Russia, it is much easier to get medication, and she feels embarrassed that she cannot be trusted to take her medications without being watched. Her biggest concerns, however, are the effects of this treatment on her job as a housekeeper. She has six clients, all Russian, and typically spends approximately 6 to 7 hours at a single home each day with the expectation that she will have completed her work before 5:00 p.m. Giving up three mornings each week would therefore disrupt the work schedules she has established with her clients and thus jeopardize her employment situation.

As the visit ends, Dr. Davies indicates that close contacts (such as family and friends) will have to be skin-tested for tuberculosis and/or obtain chest x-rays. Upon hearing this, Mrs. Rosenberg begins to weep uncontrollably.

5   Why might this request for family, friends, and other close contacts to be tested for TB be particularly upsetting to Mrs. Rosenberg?

According to the CDC, people who have had prolonged, frequent, or intense contact with a person with TB while he or she was infectious should be tested for TB. The real challenge is someone like Mrs. Rosenberg, whose pool of contacts is likely to include a fair number of individuals. Her response therefore could reflect emotions over a potential loss of privacy, shame and guilt over possibly infecting someone close to her, and fear of a possible negative response from some of her clients/employers.

> One month after Mrs. Rosenberg is diagnosed with TB and begins DOT treatment, her husband loses his job. She has been traveling 3 days a week to the Health Center to receive her medications and pays for her own transportation every single time. She wakes up very early to travel to the Health Center and does not return home until 8 p.m. six days per week, causing her employers to complain that her work has been affected. It begins to wear on her, and she is struggling with the time that it takes and the pressure to support her family. She visits Dr. Davies' office sobbing that she can't do it anymore. Again, she asks, "Why don't you trust me? Haven't I earned your trust? This is becoming very difficult for me and I need to know some other options. Can you please call the Health Department and ask if someone can come to my home?"

6   Is it possible to make alternative arrangements for Mrs. Rosenberg to receive DOT for TB at home?

It is important that DOT be carried out at times and in locations that are as convenient as possible for patients to enable completion of the recommended therapy. Mrs. Rosenberg's therapy has taken place in the Health Center. However, in most jurisdictions, arrangements can be made for DOT to occur at the patient's home. For Mrs. Rosenberg, this would significantly improve her quality of life. In some situations, staff of correctional facilities or of drug treatment programs, home health care workers, the maternal and child health staff, or designated community members can provide DOT. If the Health Center can arrange home visits three times per week by a field worker, Mrs. Rosenberg should be informed that she will be routinely asked about adherence at follow-up visits. She should expect that her pills will be counted and she may be asked to provide urine samples periodically to check for the presence of drug metabolites. She will also be re-examined frequently to assess her response to treatment and told that if her sputum remains positive after 2 months of treatment, she will continue to be monitored for the remainder of treatment. Again, using a trained Russian interpreter to explain what Mrs. Rosenberg can anticipate will improve adherence. According to the CDC, establishing a relationship with the patient and addressing barriers to adherence is the core of a successful DOT program.

References: Case 6

Aranguri C., Davidson B., Ramirez R. Patterns of communication through interpreters: a detailed sociolinguistic analysis. *J Gen Intern Med* 2006;21: 623–9.

Bass J.B. Epidemiology of tuberculosis. UpToDate 2007. Available at: http://www.uptodate.com.

Bass J.B. Treatment of latent tuberculosis infection in HIV-negative patients. UpToDate 2007. Available at: http://www.uptodate.com.

Bass J.B. Tuberculin skin testing and other tests for latent tuberculosis infection. UpToDate 2007. Available at: http://www.uptodate.com.

Blumberg H.M., Burman W.J., Chaisson R.E. American Thoracic Society/Centers for Disease Control and Prevention/Infectious Diseases Society of America: treatment of tuberculosis. *Am J Respir Crit Care Med* 2003; 167:603.

Carrillo J.E., Green A.R., Betancourt J.R. Cross-cultural primary care: a patient-based approach. *Ann Intern Med* 1999;130:829–34.

Chen A. Doctoring across the language divide. *Health Aff* 2006;25:808–13.

DeReimer K., Chin D.P., Schecter G.F., Reingold A.L. Tuberculosis among immigrants and refugees. *Arch Intern Med* 1998;158:753–60.

Dysart-Gale D. Communication, models, professionalism, and the work of medical interpreters. *Health Commun* 2005;17:91–103.

Flores G. The impact of medical interpreter services on the quality of healthcare: a systematic review. *Med Care Res Rev* 2005;62:255–99.

Hsieh E. Conflicts in how interpreters manage their roles in provider-patient interactions. *Soc Sci Med* 2006;62:721–30.

Hsieh E. Understanding medical interpreters: reconceptualizing bilingual health communication. *Health Commun* 2006;20:177–86.

Institute of Medicine, Committee on Elimination of Tuberculosis in the United States. In: Geiter L.J., ed. *Ending Neglect: The Elimination of Tuberculosis in the United States.* Washington DC, National Academy Press, 2000.

Kleinman A., Eisenberg L., Good B. Culture, illness, and care: clinical lessons from anthropological and cross-cultural research. *Ann Intern Med* 1978;88: 251–88.

Kulkarni S.P., Alexander K.P., Lytle B., Heiss G., Peterson E.D. Long-term adherence with cardiovascular drug regimens. *Am Heart J* 2006;151:185–91.

Osterberg L., Blaschke T. Adherence to medication. *N Engl J Med* 2005; 353:487–97.

Romero C.M. Using medical interpreters. *Am Fam Physician* 2004;69:2720–2.

White H.D. Adherence and outcomes: it's more than taking the pills. *Lancet* 2005;366:1989–91.

CASE 7

Isabel Delgado

A 47-year-old Dominican woman with hypertension

Debbie Salas-Lopez, MD, MPH, FACP, and Eric Gertner, MD, MPH
Lehigh Valley Hospital and Health Network, Allentown, PA, USA

Educational Objectives

- Describe approaches for obtaining a patient history in a culturally appropriate manner that includes the context of the day life of the patient.
- Identify challenges a patient may face when taking prescribed medications.
- Recognize that previous cultural and life experiences may be a part of the perception patients may have of traditional medicine.
- Describe the framework for providing cross-cultural communication.

TACCT Domains: 4, 6

Case Summary, Questions and Answers

Mrs. Isabel Delgado is a 47-year-old woman from the Dominican Republic who presents to the Emergency Department (ED) complaining of severe headaches. She has a history of chronic hypertension and her blood pressure is elevated in the ED. After ruling out life-threatening conditions, she is referred back to the residents' outpatient clinic where

Achieving Cultural Competency: A case-based approach to training health professionals,
1st edition. Edited by L Hark, H DeLisser. © 2009 Blackwell Publishing,
ISBN: 9781405180726.

she has been followed for general medical care for the past 4 years. On this day, she returns to the clinic and is seen by a medical resident who she has never met before. He asks her if she has been taking her blood pressure medication, and she answers, "Not really, only once in a while." He admonishes her to do so, stressing that she is at risk of having a stroke, or a heart attack, or developing kidney failure, and indicates that her headaches are probably caused by poorly controlled hypertension.

1   Is the resident's response likely to motivate Mrs. Delgado to take her medication on a regular basis?

Medication adherence is affected by many factors. Often it is framed strictly in terms of what the patient fails to do, and patients like Mrs. Delgado are labeled as "non-compliant." When poor patient adherence is seen only as a patient problem, this attitude can interfere with the building of a rapport between the patient and the physician. However, poor adherence also may arise from physician failures and inadequate delivery of care. To improve adherence, physicians should explore the patient's explanatory model of illness during the initial history of present illness. Although this inquiry may require a few additional minutes, it can go a long way in helping the physician understand the patient's perspective. Mrs. Delgado's explanatory model of illness for high blood pressure may be very different from that of her treating physician. If the resident had asked, he would have learned that Mrs. Delgado does not understand that high blood pressure needs to be treated every day, even in the absence of symptoms. Consequently, she believed that she needed to take her medication only if her blood pressure was high enough to cause a headache. Eliciting this information may be initiated by asking, "Mrs. Delgado, what does having high blood pressure mean to you?" (see Appendix 2).

In addition, Mrs. Delgado is frequently seen by a different resident every time she comes to the clinic. She is weary of having to repeat her story to each new resident, and so she is not very forthcoming with information. As a result, only a cursory history is usually obtained, that her level of understanding of the meaning and significance of her illness has never been fully captured by her physician. Having a constant provider at the clinic, whether it is a resident, nurse practitioner, or an attending physician, can help to alleviate this problem for many patients.

2   What other influences might affect Mrs. Delgado's decision to take her medication?

Mrs. Delgado's frame of reference about her illness may be based on what she knows about high blood pressure from newspapers or television or what it means to her family and friends. Patients often have trusting relationships with family and friends and may seek additional medical advice and/or obtain medications from them, which may be contradictory to the physician's advice. Therefore, it is important to explore with Mrs. Delgado what she has learned about high blood pressure from other sources. In fact, Mrs. Delgado left the clinic and later asked her neighbor for advice. The neighbor referred her to the local pharmacy and gave Mrs. Delgado instructions to ask for Carlos, the pharmacy technician. She told her that Carlos was very good at finding different medicines that were less expensive and over the counter.

In the local pharmacy, Mrs. Delgado explained to Carlos that she did not believe her diagnosis of high blood pressure because she usually feels fine with the exception of occasional headaches. In fact, she was feeling perfectly fine today. She went on to explain that what she really needed was to lose weight, eat better, and relax more from a stressful nighttime job. Carlos helped Mrs. Delgado, by recommending a weight loss dietary supplement, vitamins for better appetite, and something to stay awake at night while at work. Given that her neighbor had vouched for Carlos, and his apparent helpfulness, Mrs. Delgado decided to purchase the over-the-counter product instead of the medication prescribed by her physician.

3   What other social factors should be considered for Mrs. Delgado that might impact her adherence?

Life responsibilities such as work, care of children and obligations at home, and family may be significant and overwhelming and can greatly impact patient adherence to physician recommendations. Patients are not necessarily or immediately forthcoming about these social determinants of health, and thus physicians should have a low-threshold for asking about these factors. With respect to Mrs. Delgado, she works at night and takes an over-the-counter medications ("pep pill") to stay awake during work. She is reluctant to share this information with the resident. When she returns home in the early morning, her husband is on his way out to work. She must get her four children off to school and ensure they have everything they need for the day. She is not only worried about her high blood pressure, but she is also concerned about what may happen to her children if she is not well enough to work.

> One month later, Mrs. Delgado returns to the outpatient clinic for follow-up. She is seen by another resident, who determines that her blood pressure is still high. When the resident asks her if she is taking her medications daily, she says she is trying to do her best but finds that she can't always take them every day. The resident asks why, and Mrs. Delgado says that she is just too busy. The resident begins by admonishing her to take the medication daily and says that she must also follow a low-salt diet to reduce her blood pressure. Once again, Mrs. Delgado listens carefully and begins to wonder how she is going to comply with this. She returns to the clinic 1 month later and her blood pressure is still uncontrolled. She admits that she has not changed her diet.

4   In what way could the patient's cultural background be playing a role in her poor adherence?

Understanding a patient's cultural background is extremely important as it can facilitate communication and potentially strengthen the doctor–patient relationship. Mrs. Delgado came to the U.S. 10 years ago from the Dominican Republic to visit her family. She stayed in the U.S. and has never returned to the Dominican Republic. She has an expired visitor's visa and lives in fear of deportation. Even though she has lived in the U.S. for a decade, she does not understand nor accept many of the American, health beliefs, or practices and holds on to traditional cultural health beliefs and practices from the Dominican Republic. Because of her cultural background, she is also extremely respectful of physicians and therefore, when originally given the prescription for the anti-hypertensive medications, she never considered asking about side effects, costs, or mechanism of action.

Understanding that Mrs. Delgado may have different dietary practices, does not believe in taking prescribed medications, and prefers to take natural supplements and vitamins may yield a better response from the patient regarding her treatment. Physicians should take the time to ask patients about culturally relevant practices in a nonjudgmental manner, including the use of over-the-counter and other medications. Equally important, asking patients about the use of other healers or health consultants may reveal that the physician is not the only person the patient seeks health advice from (see above).

> *Mrs. Delgado returned to the clinic 3 months later, as requested by the medical resident. This time she was fortunate enough to see the same medical resident who remembered her story. When the young physician asked if she had taken the medication, Mrs. Delgado acknowledged that she had decided to purchase an over-the-counter weight loss supplement, a vitamin, and a "pep pill" to stay awake at night. The resident looked up the supplements in the Physician's Desk Reference and explained to Mrs. Delgado that they had known significant effects on blood pressure. Mrs. Delgado gave him the name of the pharmacy where she purchased it so that he could get more information. The medical resident called and asked to speak to Carlos. After explaining to Carlos the importance of the treatment of hypertension in acutely ill patients, he asked him to refrain from giving patients medical advice or substitutes for prescribed medications. Mrs. Delgado agreed to buy the prescribed medication and return to the clinic 1 month later to see him.*

5   In what way does a system of seeing a different resident at each visit adversely affecting Mrs. Delgado's health?

Lack of continuity reduces her ability to develop a relationship with a physician and promote a realistic health care plan. Residents, especially in busy clinics, focus on quantitative goals (normalize blood pressure and blood sugar levels and "doing what the physician said") as parameters of success without evaluating the qualitative aspects (how and why) of a patient's life and the context of a life she lives within. Without this latter component, the emphasis on "good numbers" does not translate to improve health outcomes. Hence, training in areas such as cultural competency and assessing health literacy are essential for effective medical interviewing.

6   Was it helpful for the medical resident to call the pharmacy to speak to Carlos?

Physicians should ask patients who else is involved in their health care. With permission, they can then engage those individuals when needed. Asking Carlos to refrain from giving medical advice is important in this case and also helps Mrs. Delgado better understand that she takes significant risk when she does not follow medical advice. Understanding who is part of the health care team is important for the physician in practice. The physician can then negotiate a mutually acceptable solution with the patient. Dr. Robert Like and his colleagues have developed the ETHNIC framework that is simple to use and remember, as shown in Table 7.1.

Table 7.1 ETHNIC: A framework for culturally competent clinical practice

E: Explanation	What do you think may be the reason you have these symptoms?
	What do friends, family and others say about these symptoms?
	Do you know anyone else who has had or who has this kind of problem?
	Have you heard about/read/seen it on TV/radio/newspaper?
	(If the patient cannot offer explanation, ask what most concerns them about their problems.)
T: Treatment	What kinds of medicines, home remedies, or other treatments have you tried for this illness?
	Is there anything you eat, drink, or do (or avoid) on a regular basis to stay healthy? Tell me about it.
	What kind of treatment are you seeking from me?
H: Healers	Have you sought any advice from alternative/folk healers, friends, or other people (non-doctors) for help with your problems? Tell me about it.
N: Negotiate	Negotiate options that will be *mutually acceptable* to you and your patient and that do not contradict, but rather incorporate your patient's beliefs.
	Ask what are the most important results your patient hopes to achieve from this intervention.
I: Intervention	Determine an intervention with your patient. May include incorporation of alternative treatments, spirituality, and healers as well as other cultural practices (e.g. foods eaten or avoided in general, and when sick).
C: Collaboration	Collaborate with the patient, family members, other health care team members, healers, and community resources.

Source: Like R.C., Steiner R.P., Rubel A.J.. Recommended core curriculum guidelines on culturally sensitive and competent healthcare. *Fam Med* 1996;28:291–7.

References: Case 7

American College of Physicians. Racial and ethnic disparities in healthcare: a position paper of the American College of Physicians. *Ann Intern Med* 2004;141(3):226–32.

Betancourt J.R. Cross-cultural medical education: conceptual approaches and frameworks for evaluation. *Acad Med 2003*;78(6):560–9.

Brach C., Fraser I. Reducing disparities through culturally competent healthcare: an analysis of the business case. *Qual Manag Healthcare* 2002;10(4):15–28.

Carrillo J.E., Green A.R., Betancourt J.R. Cross-cultural care: a patient-based approach. *Ann Intern Med* 1999;130(10):829–34.

Cooper L.A., Hill M.N., Powe N.R. Designing and evaluating interventions to eliminate racial and ethnic disparities in healthcare. *J Gen Intern Med* 2002;17(6):477–86.

Kundhal K.K. Cultural diversity: an evolving challenge to physician-patient communication. *JAMA* 2003;289(1):94.

Levin S.J., Like R.C., Gottlieb J.E. Ethnic: a framework for culturally competent clinical practice. In appendix: Useful clinical interviewing mnemonics. *Patient Care* 2000;34(9):188–9.

Like R.C., Steiner R.P., Rubel A.J. Recommended core curriculum guidelines on culturally sensitive and competent healthcare. *Fam Med* 1996;28:291–7.

Napoles-Springer A.M., Santoyo J., Houston K., Perez-Stable E.J., Stewart A.L. Patients' perceptions of cultural factors affecting the quality of their medical encounters. *Health Expect* 2005;8(1):4–17.

Tervalon M. Components of culture in health for medical students' education. *Acad Med* 2003;78(6):570–6.

Weissman J.S., Betancourt J.S., Campbell E.G., et al. Resident physicians' preparedness to provide cross-cultural care. *JAMA* 2005;294:1058–67.

CASE 8

George Dennis

A 35-year-old African American man with AIDS

Ronald G. Collman, MD
University of Pennsylvania School of Medicine, Philadelphia, PA, USA

Educational Objectives

- Explain the interface of race and sexual orientation in health care.
- Demonstrate sensitivity to cultural issues in clinical practice and employ a setting that is safe for disclosure and that ensures patient privacy.
- Describe appropriate approaches to discussing potentially sensitive and private issues with patients, to ensure nonjudgmental interactions.
- Respect patient confidentiality and autonomy, yet understand the limits to this and be able to successfully integrate family members when necessary.

TACCT Domains: 3, 6

Case Summary, Questions and Answers

George Dennis is a 35-year-old African American man who comes unaccompanied to his primary care physician (PCP), Dr. Carey, complaining of a cough for the past 7 days. In addition, he reports that, for the past 3 months, he has not been able to play his usual weekend basketball game because of shortness of breath. Given the acute cough,

---

Achieving Cultural Competency: A case-based approach to training health professionals, 1st edition. Edited by L Hark, H DeLisser. © 2009 Blackwell Publishing, ISBN: 9781405180726.

Dr. Carey believes that Mr. Dennis has a community-acquired pneumo-nia that could be treated as an outpatient. However, because of the patient's young age, as well as his shortness of breath, Dr. Carey is also concerned about HIV-related pneumonia and therefore questions him about risk factors for HIV, asking Mr. Dennis if he is "gay," a "drug user," and if he has "unprotected sex" with women. Mr. Dennis denies all three. He is given an antibiotic for a presumed community-acquired pneumonia and instructed to follow-up in 2 weeks if he does not im-prove. Mr. Dennis returns to Dr. Carey's office 1 week later, this time with his sister, who urged him to come back sooner. She reports that his cough has gotten worse and he appears to be persistently short of breath. Because of Mr. Dennis' worsening condition, Dr. Carey sends him immediately to the Emergency Department (ED). There, he is found to be hypoxemic (oxygen saturation on room air was 83%) with his chest x-ray demonstrating a diffuse interstitial pattern. He is consequently admitted to the hospital where bronchoscopy is performed and he is diagnosed with Pneumocystis jiroveci (formerly known as Pneumocystis carinii) pneumonia. Subsequent testing confirms that Mr. Dennis is HIV-positive. When questioned again about risk factors for HIV infection, Mr. Dennis acknowledges that he has engaged in same-sex activity and has had unprotected sex with other men, but that he is currently in a monogamous same-sex relationship. He agrees to notify his partner of his HIV status, but insists that this information not be disclosed in any way to members of his family.

1   Why might Mr. Dennis have been less than forthcoming about his sexual activity and sexual orientation during the initial visit?

It almost goes without saying that topics such as sexual orientation and sexual activity may be difficult for patients to discuss during an initial visit. For some it may be simply the discomfort of reveal-ing something highly personal to a stranger. Additionally, although there has been a steady increase in the acceptance of homosexuality in the wider society, individual gay men and lesbian women may still have a fear of negative consequences that might come with reveal-ing their orientation. Or they may be at a stage in which they are not yet personally comfortable with being open about their homosexu-ality. These concerns about publicly acknowledging one's sexual ori-entation may be further heightened among blacks, given that open expression of homosexuality is less accepted in the African American community. Further, many men with same-sex sexual activity may not self-identify as homosexual or gay. This occurs among all groups, but has been suggested to be more common in the African American community, where the phenomenon has been termed being on the "down low." Being on the "down low" contributes to the increasing HIV rates in African American women, as they can be partnered with a man who is having unprotected sex with men. The societal pressure on men to be on the "down low" may lead to significant stress and result in high-risk sexual practices. The media attention to this issue has not yet resulted in sufficient research support to fully investigate this behavior.

Study Shows Doctors are Often in the Dark about Patients' Sexual Behavior

The New York City Department of Health recently published a study of 452 men who were interviewed anonymously at gay bars and clubs. Participants were tested for HIV and offered medical and social services as needed. The study showed that 39% of the men who had sex with other men in New York City had not disclosed their sexual orientation to their doctors. The survey also showed that 60% of African Americans, 48% of Hispanics, and 47% of Asian men who had sex with men *did not* disclose their sexual activity compared with 19% of Caucasian men.

The study also showed that men who disclosed having sex with men were twice as likely to have been tested for HIV, compared with those who did not disclose their same-sex activity (63% vs. 36%). The low rate of HIV testing among nondisclosers suggests that health care providers continue to practice risk-based HIV testing in New York City. Therefore, health care providers may not offer HIV testing unless they know that a patient has a risk factor for HIV. The current national CDC guidelines for HIV testing advise health care providers to offer HIV testing to *all* patients between the ages of 13 and 64.

2   When exploring risk factors for HIV with patients, what approaches might be used in discussing these potentially sensitive and private issues?

Eliciting honest and complete responses around issues such as sexual orientation and sexual activity, as well as illicit activities such as drug use, may require an approach that is different from that used to obtain other parts of the medical history. Questions should be asked in a way that is as nonjudgmental as possible and in a manner that distinguishes between the behavior and the person. Asking, "Are you sexually active with other men?" is preferable to, "Are you gay?" or "You don't have sex with other men, do you?" Similarly, "Have you used any drugs that involve sharing needles?" is more likely to elicit useful information than, "You aren't a drug user, are you?" It is important to provide a setting that is safe for disclosure and ensures privacy. Family members and friends may need to be excluded from the conversation. Each situation is unique and certainly requires sensitivity and skill, so as not to alienate loved ones. Also bear in mind that probing or pushing too hard may increase the resistance of the patient, recognizing that, although the patient may not be forthcoming now, with time as trust develops they may be more willing to talk about these sensitive issues. Finally, it is important to recognize that all patients should be considered as being at risk for HIV infection, so the absence of specific identifiable factors should not exclude consideration of that diagnosis in the appropriate setting. Some HIV specialists feel that elucidating the patient's current high-risk behavior is more important than the manner of the initial transmission of the HIV infection.

The Epidemiology of HIV Infection

It is estimated that, in the U.S., about 1.2 million people are currently infected with HIV, of whom 44% acquired infection through sex between men, 34% through heterosexual intercourse, and 17% through drug injection activity. The proportion of infections in women has risen dramatically (currently ~27%), mainly through sexual acquisition. New infections acquired through blood and related products are now rare in the developed world due to excellent screening procedures. Infections among children are also now infrequent in the U.S. (<200/year) due to screening and antiretroviral treatment of pregnant women.

Racial and ethnic minorities are disproportionately affected by HIV. About 50% of the new AIDS diagnoses in the U.S. occur among African Americans, despite the fact that they represent only 12% of the U.S. population, and 20% occur among Hispanics (14% of the U.S. population). The rate of HIV/AIDS diagnosis is 7 times higher among African American men than white men, and 21 times higher among African American women than white women. Up to half of infected individuals in minority groups do not know their infection status.

Worldwide it is estimated that about 33 million people are currently infected (including 2.5 million children) with 2.5 million new infections and 2.1 million deaths each year, plus about 20 million who have already died of the infection.

> Mr. Dennis was treated with trimethoprim/sulfamethoxazole and pred-
> nisone and was discharged from the hospital after 8 days. During his
> hospitalization, his biological family did not learn of the exact nature
> of his infection, believing instead that he had a routine pneumonia.
> He was referred to the immunodeficiency clinic where he was found
> to have a CD4 count of 100 and a plasma viral load of 150,000, and
> was started on three-drug HAART (highly active antiretroviral therapy)
> treatment. When seen 4 months later, his immune status had improved
> significantly, with his viral load declining to undetectable levels and his
> CD4 count rising to 350. Mr. Dennis reminded the physician again that
> he did not want his family to know of his AIDS diagnosis. He informed
> the physician that he had designated his partner, Mark Barnes, as his
> surrogate decision maker and the only one with whom the physicians
> could discuss his medical issues.

3   How might you respond to Mr. Dennis when he asks you to withhold information from family members?

Patient autonomy and confidentiality are fundamental patient rights
that should be respected and protected as best as possible. In addition to these ethical constraints, disclosure of confidential patient
information is legally restricted under the federal law, "Health Insurance Portability and Accountability Act of 1996" (HIPAA), which
regulates how personal health information is handled and gives individuals the right to restrict access to that information. This would of
course be especially relevant for highly sensitive information, such
as a diagnosis of HIV/AIDS. HIPAA regulations do not restrict sharing of medical information necessary to provide appropriate medical
care. In addition, HIPAA regulations generally also allow information to be shared with family members unless patients indicate that
they do not want it disclosed. Nevertheless, if a patient asks that the
information not be shared, it is incumbent on the physician and all
health care providers to follow those instructions, particularly when
an alternate surrogate is identified (Mr. Barnes).

However, in Mr. Dennis' case, the reality is that he is asking the
physician to make a promise that may be difficult to keep. The information he is trying to conceal from his family may eventually
become known to them, either inadvertently or through their own
deductive reasoning. In other circumstances, where an alternative

surrogate decision maker has not been identified, disclosure may be required because the family must become involved due to issues related to care or decision making. Concealment also has the potential of undermining the family's trust in the physician if they discover that information has been withheld from them, even at the instruction of the patient. Further, anecdotal experience suggests that most families do want to be involved in the care of a loved one and do respond well when they learn that a loved one is HIV-positive.

> *Six months after his discharge, Mr. Dennis was admitted to the hospital with jaundice and altered mental status (obtundation) that was believed to be the result of liver toxicity from the HAART. His partner, Mark Barnes, acting as his decision maker, instructed the medical team not to inform Mr. Dennis' family of his admission. He believed this was consistent with the wishes of the patient. Five days after his admission, Mr. Dennis' sister and mother learned that he was in the hospital and arrived there, extremely angry that they had not been immediately informed of his hospital admission. They confronted Mr. Dennis' nurse, demanding to speak to Dr. Carey about why the family had not been notified of Mr. Dennis' admission and why medical decisions regarding the care of their brother and son were being made without their involvement.*

4 How might Dr. Carey respect the patient's autonomy while responding meaningfully to the family?

There may well be several possible responses, but based on our experience, we believe that advocating for disclosure is most helpful in both the short and long term. If, as in this case, the patient is not able to participate in further discussions, the process may begin by first meeting with Mr. Dennis' partner (Mr. Barnes) and expressing the concerns of the medical team about further concealment of the HIV/AIDS diagnosis and continued exclusion of the family from discussions. It would be important to convey to Mr. Barnes that: (i) the current situation, and the tension that has arisen, distract the physicians and nurses from their care of Mr. Dennis; (ii) it is in the best interest of the patient, given this distraction, to inform the family; and (iii) ideally, Mr. Barnes should be part of this conversation. Here is an example of the language that may be helpful:

> *"We are at a point now where, in practical terms, it is impossible for us to continue to keep his diagnosis a secret from his family. More importantly, the efforts we make to conceal his diagnosis and his sexual*

orientation from the family are distracting us from providing the best care possible for Dennis. I hope that you and I together can figure out the best way of informing the family so that we can diffuse any hurt or anger they may be feeling and to gain their support for Dennis."

If Mr. Barnes, acting as Mr. Dennis' surrogate, agrees, Dr. Carey should then meet with the family, ideally with Mr. Barnes present. After revealing the diagnosis, the family should be informed of Mr. Dennis' previous wishes that his HIV status not be disclosed to family and that he had designated Mr. Barnes to make decisions for him if he could not speak for himself. This will help the family to understand the professional and legal obligations that led to withholding information from family members and deferring to Mr. Barnes for medical decisions. The family may well feel hurt, anger, or embarrassment about learning of the diagnosis and/or that their son/brother had chosen to exclude them. It is important that these emotions, if present, be acknowledged and discussed.

"Let me begin by saying that Mr. Dennis has AIDS. We made this diagnosis six months ago when he was hospitalized for pneumonia. At that time, and then subsequently, he gave clear instructions that his family not be informed about his disease. Although I was not in agreement with this, my professional obligations require that I do my best to protect his privacy. However, I had made it clear to Mr. Dennis that there might come a time in the future when it would be best for us to speak to you as we are doing now. He had also legally selected Mr. Barnes as the person to make decisions for him if he could not speak for himself. This is why you were not involved in his decision making. I suspect that you are feeling several emotions right now. The diagnosis may be a shock to you and/or there may be some anger or hurt that George had chosen to conceal this information from you. What are you feeling right now?"

The meeting should conclude, ideally, with a sense of an alliance of all involved to do what is best for the patient's recovery. Should Mr. Barnes refuse Dr. Carey's suggestions, regardless of how challenging it is for him, Dr. Carey must respect the patient's wishes. Often in medicine, respecting autonomy of the patient can be painful; watching a 20-year-old man with three small children die of anemia due to refusal of blood transfusions, or the inability to bring a family together over an illness can be challenging for all physicians.

Fundamentally, our patient's bodies and choices are theirs and doing no harm includes respecting wishes we may not choose for
ourselves.

References: Case 8

Bernstein K.T., Liu K.L., Begier E.M., Koblin B., Karpati A., Murrill C. Same-
sex attraction disclosure to health care providers among New York City
men who have sex with men: implications for HIV testing approaches.
Arch Intern Med 2008;168(13):1458–64.

Centers for Disease Control and Prevention (CDC). HIV prevalence, un-
recognized infection, and HIV testing among men who have sex with
men–five U.S. cities, June 2004-April 2005. *MMWR Morb Mortal Wkly Rep*
2005;54(24):597–601.

Denizet-Lewis B. Doubles lives on the down low. *New York Times*, August 3,
2003.

Hook M.K., Cleveland J.L. To tell or not to tell: breaching confidentiality
with clients with HIV and AIDS. *Ethics Behav* 1999;9:365–81.

Martinez J., Hosek S.G. An exploration of the down-low identity: non gay-
identified young African-American men who have sex with men. *J Natl
Med Assoc* 2005;97(8):1103–12.

Meckler G.D., Elliott M.N., Kanouse D.E., Beals K.P., Schuster M.A. Nondis-
closure of sexual orientation to a physician among a sample of gay, lesbian,
and bisexual youth. *Arch Pediatr Adolesc Med* 2006;160:1248–54.

Miller M., Serner M., Wagner M. Sexual diversity among black men who
have sex with men in an inner-city community. *J Urban Health* 2005;82(1):
i26–34 (suppl 1).

Gerberding J.L. Clinical practice. Occupational exposure to HIV in healthcare
settings. *N Engl J Med* 2003;348(9):826–33.

Gostin L.O. National health information privacy: regulations under the
Health Insurance Portability and Accountability Act. *JAMA* 2001;285(23):
3015–21.

Lehman D.A., Farquhar C. Biological mechanisms of vertical human immunodeficiency virus (HIV-1) transmission. *Rev Med Virol* 2007;17(6):381–403.

Lo B., Dornbrand L., Dubler N.N. HIPAA and patient care: the role for professional judgment. *JAMA* 2005;293(14):1766–71.

Malebranche D.J., Peterson J.L., Fullilove R.E., Stackhouse R.W. Race and
sexual identity: perceptions about medical culture and healthcare among
black men who have sex with men. *J Natl Med Assoc* 2004;96(1):97–
107.

Rabow M.W., Hauser J.M., Adams J. Supporting family caregivers at the end
of life: "they don't know what they don't know." *JAMA* 2004;291(4):483–
91.

Stokes J.P., Peterson J.L. Homophobia, self-esteem, and risk for HIV among African American men who have sex with men. *AIDS Educ Prev* 1998; 10(3):278–92.

UNAIDS/WHO AIDS Epidemic Update: December 2007. World Health Organization, Geneva, Switzerland.

Vernillo A.T., Wolpe P.R., Halpern S.D. Re-examining ethical obligations in the intensive care unit: HIV disclosure to surrogates. *Crit Care* 2007;11:125.

Wawer M.J., Gray R.H., Sewankambo N.K., et al. Rates of HIV-1 transmission per coital act, by stage of HIV-1 infection, in Rakai, Uganda. *J Infect Dis* 2005; 191(9):1403–9.

Young R.M., Meyer I.H. The trouble with "MSM" and "WSW": erasure of the sexual-minority person in public health discourse. *Am J Public Health* 2005;95:1144–9.

CASE 9

Mary Jones

A 2-year-old Caucasian girl with delayed speech development

Dodi Meyer, MD, Hetty Cunningham, MD, Rica Mauricio,
and Alexandra Schieber

Columbia University College of Physicians and Surgeons, New York, NY, USA

Educational Objectives

- Describe the four domains of the social context review of systems.
- Define an approach for exploring a "differential diagnosis" of nonadherence.
- Identify the indicators of a low level of literacy.
- Describe the relationship between health literacy, health outcomes, and medication errors.

TACCT Domains: 1, 4

Case Summary, Questions and Answers

Mary is a 2-year-old Caucasian girl who comes to the community-based primary care clinic with her mother (Ms. Jones) for her well child care visit. She is seen by her pediatrician, Dr. Robinson. During the routine developmental screening, Dr. Robinson queries the mother about the number of words that Mary can say and about her ability to put two words together. Ms. Jones reports that Mary only speaks two words

Achieving Cultural Competency: A case-based approach to training health professionals,
1st edition. Edited by L Hark, H DeLisser. © 2009 Blackwell Publishing,
ISBN: 9781405180726.

> other than "mommy" and "daddy." Mary's physical exam is normal and she has no other abnormalities. Her gross and fine motor skills are normal. Records show that Mary also passed her universal newborn hearing screening test. Dr. Robinson explains to Ms. Jones that Mary has delayed speech development. She suggests that Mary be referred to the Early Intervention Program for evaluation of the speech problem and for coordination of speech therapy. She also recommends that Mary's hearing be retested. Dr. Robinson calls Early Intervention while the mother is in the office and tells Ms. Jones that Early Intervention will call her at home to set up an appointment. Before leaving the clinic, the front desk makes an appointment for a hearing evaluation at a specialty office elsewhere in the city and gives the mother a slip with this information. Ms. Jones is also given a follow-up appointment with Dr. Robinson in 1 month. Mom seems very concerned, says "thank you," and appears to understand.

1 What additional information might have been helpful to Dr. Robinson in developing a plan of action for Mary and her family?

In order to assess a patient's ability to follow-up with any clinical recommendation, their social context needs to be explored. To gain understanding of factors that may impact on a patient's ability to adhere to recommendations, we suggest using the "Four Domains of the Social Context" "Review of Systems" described by Green and coworkers, as shown in Table 9.1. Similar to the traditional review of systems, these questions are used selectively in a focused, problem-oriented manner. In this case, the following questions would be helpful:

• Where does Ms. Jones live?
• What is her economic status and employment situation? (If she works during the day, is there someone who can answer the phone and schedule an appointment?)
• Can she take a day from work to take her daughter to a hearing test? If not, does she have a support network?
• What is her literacy level? (Can she follow written instructions on how to get to the hospital?)
• Are there significant stresses in her life that may affect her ability to follow through with the plan? Important sources of stress in patients' lives include the other factors described in the list (i.e., financial problems, housing problems, new environments, etc.) as well as domestic violence, substance abuse, family conflict, and crime, among a multitude of others.

Table 9.1 The Four Domains of the Social Context "Review of Systems"*

Social stressors and support network

What is causing the most stress in your life? How do you deal with this?[†]

Do you have friends or relatives that you can call on for help? Do they live with you or close by?

Are you very involved in a religious or social group?

Do you feel that God (or spirituality) provides a strong source of support in your life?

Change of environment

Where are you from originally? When did you come to this (country, city, town)?

What made you decide to come to this (country, city, town)?

How have you found life here compared with life in your (country, city, town)?

What was medical care like there compared with here?

Life control

Do you ever feel that you're not able to afford food, medications, and/or medical expenses, ?[†]

How do you keep track of appointments/medications?

Are you more concerned about how your health affects you right now, or how it might affect you in the future?

Do you feel that you have the ability to affect your own health (or particular medical condition) or is it out of your control?

Do you ever feel that you are treated unfairly by the health care system for any reason (e.g. socioeconomic status, insurance status, race/ethnicity, language, etc.)?[†]

Literacy

Is understanding or reading your medicine bottles' instructions or other patient information difficult for you?

Do you have trouble with reading in general?[†]

---

*This list presents examples of questions in four major domains of social-context analysis. Exploration of these domains can be helpful for all patients, but particularly so for non-majority patients, and is a necessary complement to exploration of cross-cultural domains.

[†]This is one of a number of questions that may be particularly difficult for patients to discuss openly. It may be helpful to preface the question with a statement of normalization, e.g. "I find that many people have trouble reading the complicated instructions that doctor's give out. Have you had trouble with this?"

Source: Green A.R., Betancourt J.R., Carrillo J.E. Integrating social factors into cross-cultural medical education. *Acad Med* 2002;77:193–7.

Unfortunately, Dr. Robinson did not go through these questions during this visit. In many instances, when there are pressing "medical" issues, providers overlook the social context due to time pressures; alternatively, they may not appreciate the value of these types of questions. Ultimately, investing the time in obtaining this information up front often proves to be crucial in creating a partnership between physician and patient, which in turn increases physician understanding, facilitates patients' adherence, and improves health outcomes.

Universal Newborn Hearing Evaluation

Significant hearing loss is one of the most common major abnormalities present at birth and, if undetected, impedes speech, language, and cognitive development. In 1999, the American Academy of Pediatrics recommended the development of national universal newborn hearing screening programs. This policy establishes benchmarks to ensure that all newborns with hearing loss are identified prior to hospital discharge or before 3 months of age. Early detection of hearing loss coupled with early intervention has been shown to maximize the development of linguistic and literacy skills, cognition, reading, and social emotional development.

Early Intervention

The Early Intervention Program is part of a national effort initiated by Congress in 1986 through the passage of the Individuals with Disabilities Education Act (Public Law 99-457). The law created an entitlement to a wide range of rehabilitative services for infants and toddlers from birth through age 2. Early Intervention is a comprehensive interagency program that supports infants and children with developmental delays through provision of needed therapies and case coordination. As a federal entitlement program, these services are universally available at no cost to the family.

One month later, Ms. Jones and Mary return to the office for their follow-up visit. Dr. Robinson asks if Mary's hearing has been tested, and Ms. Jones says she did not go to the hearing appointment. When asked why, she said that she was working and was unable to take time off to go to the appointment. When questioned whether the Early Intervention Program had called, Ms. Jones said that no one had contacted her. At this visit, Ms. Jones seems most concerned about Mary's fever, runny nose, and ear pain. Dr. Robinson's physical exam reveals that Mary has an ear infection, and she prescribes an antibiotic suspension. Dr. Robinson instructs Ms. Jones to give Mary 1 teaspoon of the antibiotic, 2 times per day for 10 days. Ms. Jones nods and seems to understand. Dr. Robinson informs Ms. Jones that the hearing test needs to be rescheduled and that she will re-refer Mary to Early Intervention. Ms. Jones is instructed to return to the clinic in 1 month for follow-up and she agrees. After the visit, Dr. Robinson wonders why Ms. Jones did not follow-up and calls Early Intervention to investigate. They explain that they tried to reach Ms. Jones several times, but were unsuccessful by phone. They sent two follow-up letters instructing her to schedule an appointment, but she never did. Dr. Robinson requests that these letters be faxed to the office for verification.

2   At this second visit, what are the potential reasons that Ms. Jones did not call Early Intervention to schedule an appointment for her child to have the hearing test?

When a patient does not follow through on previously discussed recommendations and agreed upon scheduled appointments, a provider should initiate a model of patient centered interviewing to assess the patient's perspective on the issue. This model allows a provider to explore nonadherence in a nonjudgmental way. When teaching, we refer to this process as developing a differential diagnosis of noncompliance.

We have adapted the Transtheoretical Model for behavior change as shown in Table 9.2 to help identify where the patient is in his/her thinking and to guide the clinician's efforts. Based on this model, Ms. Jones appears to acknowledge that Mary's speech is different from other children and to accept that this is a problem that needs to be addressed. Furthermore, she has expressed a desire for help. However, it would have been helpful for Dr. Robinson to explore her understanding and motivations in more detail.

Ms. Jones returns to the clinic with Mary 1 month later as scheduled. Ms. Jones explains that Mary's cold and ear pain have resolved. However, when Dr. Robinson asks if Mary took the antibiotic for all 10 days, Ms. Jones responds: "Yes. But it was hard to give the medicine in the ear, because the drops kept rolling out." When Ms. Jones is asked about the Early Intervention appointment, she says, "They never called."

Table 9.2 Using the Transtheoretical Model to explore nonadherence

---

- **Does the patient identify the issue (behavior)?**
  (Does the mother think that her child talks less than other children?)
- **Does the patient identify a problem?**
  (Does the mother think there is anything wrong with the child's speech development compared with other children her age?)
- **Does the patient desire a change?**
  (Does the mother wish to get help for her child's speech delay?)
- **Does the patient feel confident that he or she can make a change?**
  (Explore the barriers to obtaining the services.)
- **Finally, if the patient is ready, give advice and facilitate an appointment for the patient to make the change.**

Source: Prochaska J.O., Norcross J.C., DiClemente C.C. *Changing for Good*. William Morrow, New York, 1994.

3 What does Ms. Jones' confusion about giving oral medication in the ear indicate?

The improper placement of liquid antibiotic into the ear, instead of the mouth, indicates that Ms. Jones has trouble comprehending dosing instructions; either the medication instructions were improperly given/read or they were not read at all. At this point, it is important to consider the patient's health literacy level. According to *Healthy People 2010*, health literacy is defined as "the degree to which individuals have the capacity to obtain, understand, and process basic health information and services needed to make appropriate health decisions." Studies have demonstrated that individuals with low health literacy have poor health status, communication problems with providers, poor knowledge of their disease states and medication regimens, increased hospitalizations, and problems with medication adherence. The ability to read medication labels and follow their instructions, to fill out insurance forms, and to navigate the medical system all require high levels of reading and numerical skills.

To address these problems, specific communication tools have been developed and demonstrated to be effective in improving patients' understanding of medication instructions and prescribed treatments. Two highly regarded and well-evaluated communication tools are: the "Teach Back Method" and visual aids/pictorials. When using the Teach Back (or Playback) Method, the provider asks the patient to restate in his/her own words the directions that have just been given. This method encourages the clinician to take responsibility for the patient's understanding of instructions. In this case, Dr. Robinson might have asked:

"In order to make sure that I explained this to you well, could you please tell me how you are going to give this medication to Mary?"

Not surprisingly, literature has also shown that, when pictorials are combined with written or oral instructions, patient understanding of how to take medications is increased. Finally, limiting the quantity of information given at each clinical interaction and repeating instructions are always useful in improving understanding.

One month later, when Ms. Jones and Mary return for their fourth visit, Dr. Robinson asks about the referrals. Mary's mother again denies being contacted by Early Intervention. Dr. Robinson asks her if she thinks her daughter's speech delay is important and if she is concerned. After Ms. Jones states that she is very concerned, Dr. Robinson asks screening questions to elicit evidence of maternal depression or domestic violence, responses to which are both negative. Dr. Robinson hands the mother the letter she received from Early Intervention via fax. When Dr. Robinson asks the mother to read the letter, Ms. Jones says she doesn't have her glasses. Dr. Robinson then looks at the chart registration form completed by Ms. Jones on her initial visit to the clinic. She notes that the form is incomplete and contains many spelling errors; this causes her to suspect that Ms. Jones may be illiterate. She then asks Ms. Jones, "Do you feel comfortable reading this letter?" Ms. Jones replies, "No."

On further exploration, Ms. Jones reveals that she works from 7 a.m. to 7 p.m. and has no answering machine, so she never received the phone messages from Early Intervention. Dr. Robinson suspects that, in addition to her inability to read, Ms. Jones may not be able to read the bus and subway maps necessary to go to the audiologist's office. Armed with this information, she assigns an office staff member to reschedule Mary's Early Intervention and audiology appointments and to teach Ms. Jones how to get there by public transportation.

---

4 Why did it take 4 months and four visits to learn that Ms. Jones cannot read?

Health professionals rarely screen for illiteracy. Providers often associate illiteracy with poor, immigrant patients who do not speak English. Because Ms. Jones is not physically or demographically identified as an immigrant or non-English speaker, Dr. Robinson did not initially consider illiteracy. In fact, she may have been uncomfortable asking about reading ability because she did not want to insult her patient, thus jeopardizing the doctor–patient relationship.

There have been a number of studies that have evaluated providers' ability to identify illiteracy in their patients. For example, in one study, doctors correctly identified only one-third of their patients with low literacy. Not surprisingly, illiterate patients are often adept at hiding their inability to read. One study asked patients in a public hospital who had difficulty reading, "Who knows you have difficulty reading?" Sixty-seven percent of these patients never told their spouses, 19% had never told anyone, and more than 75% said they had never brought anyone who could read with them to the hospital or doctor's office.

According to the Institute of Medicine, nearly half of all American adults, 90 million, have difficulty understanding and acting upon health information. Examples of illiteracy can be seen in populations beyond immigrants and U.S.-born citizens and across boundaries of race, socioeconomic status, age, and sex. Because nonreaders tend to hide their handicap very well, health care providers and health care facilities often fail to notice, if they are looking for it at all. Special care to screening and attention must be given to patients who cannot read so that they, together with their providers, can take control of their health and the health of their families. Strategies must be put in place to assist in the identification of illiterate patients as they present for care so that their providers can deliver appropriate, efficient, and high-quality health care.

5   How can patients who have low literacy be identified?

As noted above, it can be very difficult to identify patients with inadequate literacy because of embarrassment over the subject. Table 9.3 lists indicators of low literacy level, and Table 9.4 lists direct approaches for identifying low literacy levels.

6   How could this case have been handled better to improve understanding and address patients with inadequate literacy?

Health care systems need to develop processes and multiple points to identify truly illiterate patients as they enter the medical setting. Had Ms. Jones' illiteracy been identified when she presented for care, Dr. Robinson would have spent significantly less time on this issue, and the child's receipt of needed services would have been expedited.

During the family's first and second visits, the quality of care provided by Dr. Robinson would have been improved had she explored

Table 9.3 Indicators of low literacy level

- Registration forms are filled out incorrectly or are illegible.
- Health questionnaires are skipped.
- Appointments are frequently missed.
- Frequent medication errors.
- The patient cannot name the medications he/she takes, is unable to explain why the medication was prescribed, or when and how to take it.
- The patient has memorized instructions and can repeat them, but cannot answer questions such as when a refill is needed or when the last dose was taken.
- Patients identify their medications by opening the bottles and looking at the pills rather than looking at the label.
- Lack of follow-through with referrals, imaging, and laboratory testing.
- Patients' reports of medication compliance not consistent with objective laboratory evidence.
- Patients say, "Oh, I forgot my glasses," or "I want to take this [written material] home to discuss with my wife/husband/children" rather than reviewing it with the clinician.
- Absence of newspapers, books, or magazines in the home.

Source: Carroll N. *Health Literacy: A Prescription to End Confusion*. Institute of Medicine, National Acadamies Press, Washington DC, 2004.

the social context. In her review, she might have elicited the many barriers to care: illiteracy, lack of ability to navigate public transportation, long work hours, and lack of an answering machine. Providers,who are inevitably rushed do not always have time to follow the lines of questioning suggested in this case. Frequently, during subsequent visits, when a patient returns without having followed a plan of care, providers have additional opportunities

Table 9.4 Strategies for identifying low literacy level

- Show an empty pill bottle to the patient and say: "This isn't your medicine, but if it was, how would you take it?"
- Tell a patient you would like to test their vision and give them a simple pamphlet or vision test card, starting with very large letters. If they say they forgot their glasses, be wary.

Source: Kuehn K.C. *Quick Ways to Recognize and Cope with Illiteracy*. American College of Physicians, April 2000.

to engage and access tools essential to delivery of quality care to vulnerable patients.

Finally, the key to high-quality patient care is patient-centered communication characterized by emphasis on respectful, active, nonjudgmental listening skills, and exploration of a patients' understanding, desire, and ability to follow through on clinical management plans.

Motivational interviewing technique is a communication strategy that has been shown to be effective in helping patients modify addictive behaviors and is increasingly being applied in a variety of clinical settings. The goal of motivational interviewing is to understand what the motivational state of the client is at the time and to act appropriately.

Motivational Interviewing Techniques

Motivational interviewing is characterized by eliciting motivation from the client, not trying to impose it from the outside. It has been defined as a directive, client-centered counseling style for eliciting behavior change by helping clients to explore and resolve ambivalence. Resolving ambivalence is a key to motivational interviewing.

When people move into the contemplation stage, when they are thinking about changing vs. not changing, balancing out the pros and cons, they are more susceptible to real change. However, a helping professional who starts pushing behavior change at the client at this stage will meet resistance. It is the client's task, not the counselor's, to identify and resolve his or her ambivalence. What the client needs at this point is help listing pros and cons and a nonjudgmental, encouraging professional who really listens. The client determines whether their current behavior is consistent with their goals and then makes choices to move him or herself.

The counseling style is generally a quiet, supportive, and eliciting one. In this setting, effective patient education requires more active listening than talking. The therapeutic relationship is more like a partnership than one of expert/recipient, and good provider–client rapport is crucial for success. To complement motivational interviewing-based interviews, confidence and importance rating scales are often useful. The scales are used during or at the end of the visit, when a provider might ask: "On a scale of 1 to 10, how important do you feel it is to follow the plan we discussed?" (For example: to take this medicine or to go to this appointment)"And how confident do you feel that you can do this?" (For example: remember to avoid these foods or find your way to the appointment).

Health Literacy and Assessment Tools

Health literacy is a growing concern in the U.S. Approximately 25% of the U.S. adult population cannot understand written materials that require basic reading proficiency. The Institute of Medicine has found that 40 million people have trouble linking information from that found on a dosage table to instructions provided by their physician. In a study of patients at two public hospitals, investigators found that between 24.3% and 58.2% of patients did not understand directions to take medication on an empty stomach. In comparison to those with adequate health literacy skills, patients with low health literacy skills are more susceptible to hospitalizations, many of which are due to medication errors.

Patients with inadequate health literacy often encounter numerous obstacles when navigating the health care system. Before even meeting with a health care provider, patients may struggle with tasks such as scheduling an appointment, directions to the physician's office, insurance forms, and clinic registration forms. Upon meeting with a physician, patients are often bombarded with pamphlets or explanations loaded with medical jargon. And many patients feel that their physicians spend little time explaining medical conditions. Studies estimate that medication nonadherence costs about $100 billion annually in the U.S. and accounts for 10% of hospital admissions.

Health care providers should be conscientious about the accessibility of health-related information they provide to patients. A sizable amount of health-related materials are written at a 10th grade level or higher. However, most adults read at an 8th or 9th grade level. One tool medical entities can use to assess the readability of health-related text is the SMOG Readability Formula. The SMOG Formula was created to assess the reading level required to read written work. The formula is developed on the basis of counting words of more than three syllables, taking the square root of the resulting number, and adding three. The subsequent numerical result of the formula corresponds to the appropriate grade level. A second tool to assess grade level of written materials is the Flesch-Kincaid Scale, which is included in many word processing software programs. Finally, providers should strive to use plain language, not medical jargon, when speaking with their patients.

Many health literacy experts advocate that health care entities should: (1) routinely assess literacy levels of patients and (2) distribute only health care material written at a low literacy level. We suggest three tools to assess patients' literacy levels: the Rapid Estimate of Adult Literacy in Medicine (REALM), the Test of Functional Health Literacy in Adults (TOFHLA), and the Newest Vital Sign. The REALM test was developed as a quick estimate of reading level in a medical context and takes 2 to 3 minutes to perform. In theory, the REALM would be a viable method to assess literacy, but in some environments even this short test is difficult to apply. The TOFHLA test assesses both reading comprehension and numeracy skills but is lengthy at 22 minutes. The Newest Vital Sign (NVS) involves a nutrition label, six questions, and takes 3 minute to administer. More importantly, unlike the TOFHLA, the NVS is short, and unlike the REALM, the NVS can be used on both English- and Spanish-speaking patients.

References: Case 9

American Academy of Pediatrics Task Force on Newborn and Infant Hearing Policy Statement. Newborn and infant hearing loss: detection and intervention. *Pediatrics* 1999;103(2):527–30.

Andrus M.R., Roth M.T. Health literacy: a review. *Pharmacotherapy* 2002; 22(3):282–302.

Busey S., Meurer J.R., Schum T.R. Parental perceptions of well-child care visits in an inner-city clinic. *Arch Pediatr Adolesc Med* 2002;156:62–6.

Carrillo J.E., Green A.R., Betancourt J.R. Cross-cultural primary care: a patient-based approach. *Ann Intern Med* 1999;130:829–34.

Carroll N. *Health Literacy: A Prescription to End Confusion.* Institute of Medicine, National Acadamies Press, Washington DC, 2004.

Erickson S.J., Gerstle M., Feldstein S.W. Brief interventions and motivational interviewing with children, adolescents, and their parents in pediatric healthcare settings: a review. *Arch Pediatr Adolesc Med* 2005;159:1173–80.

Green A.R., Betancourt J.R., Carrillo J.E. Integrating social factors into cross-cultural medical education. *Acad Med* 2002;77:193–7.

Kefalides P.T. Illiteracy: the silent barrier to healthcare. *Ann Intern Med* 1999;130:333–6.

Kuehn K.C. Quick ways to recognize and cope with illiteracy. American College of Physicians, April 2000.

Mika V.S., Wood P.R., Weiss B.D. Ask Me 3: improving communication in a Hispanic pediatric outpatient clinic. *Am J Health Behav* 2003;31:s115–21 (suppl 1).

Miller W.R., Rollnick S. *Motivational Interviewing: Preparing People for Change,* 2nd ed. Guilford Publishing, New York, 2002.

Powell E.C., Tanz R.R., Uyeda A., Gaffney M.B., Sheehan K.M. Injury prevention education using pictorial information. *Pediatrics* 2000;105:e16.

Prochaska J.O., Norcross J.C., DiClemente C.C. *Changing for Good.* William Morrow, New York, 1994.

Safeer R.S., Keenan J. Health literacy: the gap between physicians and patients. *Am Fam Physician* 2005;72:463–8.

Sindelar H.A., Abrantes A.M., Hart C. Motivational interviewing in pediatric practice. *Curr Probl Pediatr Adolesc Healthcare* 2004;322–39.

U.S. Department of Health and Human Services, Health Communication. *Healthy People 2010*, 2nd ed. U.S. Government Printing Office, Washington DC, 2000.

Vermiere E., Hearnshaw H., Vanroyer D., Denekens J. Adherence to treatment: 3 decades of research. *J Clin Pharmacol Ther* 2003;26:331–42.

Weiss B.D., Coyne C. Communicating with patients who cannot read. *N Engl J Med* 1997;337:272–4.

Weiss B.D., Mays M.Z., Martz W., et al. Quick assessment of literacy in primary care: the newest vital sign. *Ann Fam Med* 2005;3(6):514–22.

Williams M.V., Davis T., Parker R.M., Weiss B.D. The role of health literacy in patient-physician communication. *Fam Med* 2002;34(5):383–9.

Wilson J.F. The crucial link between literacy and health. *Ann Intern Med* 2003;139:1.

Zimmerman G.L., Olsen C.G., Bosworth M.F. A 'stages of change' approach to helping patients change behavior. *Am Fam Physician* 2000;61:1409–16.

CASE 10

Priya Krishnamurthy

A 73-year-old South Asian Indian woman with a stroke

Scott Kasner, MD, Roy Hamilton, MD, MS, Steven Messé, MD and Sashank Prasad, MD

University of Pennsylvania School of Medicine, Philadelphia, PA, USA

Educational Objectives

- Appreciate that interpretation from one language to another can impair the assessment of cognitive and language disorders.
- Remember that alternative medical treatments are encountered in nearly all cultures and may conflict with standard (Western) medical care.
- Take into account that cultural values regarding the elderly may affect decisions about long-term care.
- Predict that decisions regarding end-of-life care are influenced by numerous factors, including age, religion, and ethnicity.

TACCT Domains: 2, 4, 5, 6

Case Summary, Questions and Answers

Priya Krishnamurthy is a 73-year-old South Asian Indian woman with a history of hypertension who presents to the Emergency Department (ED) with her family because they notice she has been

Achieving Cultural Competency: A case-based approach to training health professionals, 1st edition. Edited by L Hark, H DeLisser. © 2009 Blackwell Publishing, ISBN: 9781405180726.

> bumping into objects on her right side since awakening in the morning. They claim she was not aware of this problem. An urgent CT scan is performed, which demonstrates an evolving stroke involving the left occipital lobe. Her exam reveals confusion, inattention, and some general slowing of her cognition and speech. The patient does not speak English, so her family speaks for her.

1   What impact might her inability to speak English have on the patient's evaluation?

Many individuals of Indian heritage speak English. However, it is not uncommon for elderly patients who have immigrated to the U.S. to primarily speak their indigenous languages and use their children as interpreters. (She speaks Tamil and minimal English, but mostly relies on her son to interpret for her.) This can be particularly problematic in the assessment of cognitive and aphasic disorders because the family may paraphrase the patient's speech rather than simply translate it, and may also make the patient seem better than she really is. Therefore, requesting a professional medical interpreter can be especially helpful. (On the other hand, family members may be more attuned to deviations from a patient's baseline that an interpreter might not be aware of.)

2   Although her age puts her at risk for neurovascular disease, what other factors may be influencing her confusion?

At least two factors can be cited. First, adoption of new familial roles and adaptation to a new society typically present significant challenges for older immigrants. The more disparate the culture, the greater the likelihood that the adjustment process will be difficult for the newcomer, especially the elderly. The conflicts and demands that arise from this can be particularly challenging for individuals who immigrated late in life, and thus can be a source of great stress with deleterious effects on the senior's physical and mental well-being. In addition, the perception that cognitive deficits are a normal component of aging is a common bias that may delay prompt diagnosis and treatment of emerging patterns of dementia, both on the part of patients and their families, as well as health care providers. As an elderly Asian Indian woman, she is at greater risk of coronary artery disease (CAD) than an elderly white woman.

3   What other factors in her personal and social history would be helpful to know in caring for this patient?

Given the patient's immigrant and non-Western background, it is important to have some understanding of her cultural origin as well as to inquire about her family, current living arrangements, educational background, and language skills. By using nonintrusive and carefully targeted questions, the physician learned the following:

> *Mrs. Krishnamurthy is originally from Madras (Chennai), India, and her family is Hindu. She has been widowed for 6 years, and in that time has been living with her 47-year-old son Rajan (Raj) and his family in the U.S. Raj is a software engineer for a successful company; his wife Lata is finishing her doctoral dissertation in physical chemistry; and they have two children, Rajeev and Pushpa (ages 9 and 4). Mrs. Krishnamurthy also has a daughter, Vijaya, who lives in a town 20 minutes away and is a pulmonologist at a community hospital. Mrs. Krishnamurthy does not manage her own finances or drive, and does not cook most meals, although she has in the past. Her son had always considered performing these tasks as part of his role as a good child, regardless of his mother's ability to do them. He therefore does not know for certain whether his mother would be capable of performing these activities on her own. When pressed further, he states that he has noticed that her thinking has been "off," but felt that this was normal for persons of her age.*

Hinduism

Regarded as the world's oldest religion, many of Hinduism's texts and symbols can be traced to the Indus River Valley of what is now Pakistan. Today, Hinduism has become the main religion of India, Nepal, and much of South and Southeast Asia. This spread has allowed it to become the world's third largest religion, with 13% of the global population identifying themselves as Hindus. In North America, the Hindu population exceeds one million, a number that has increased significantly since 1990.

In contrast to the three major monotheistic faiths (Christianity, Islam, and Judaism) Hinduism involves the worship of multiple deities, does not rely on a centralized structure, and is not based on the teachings of a single founder or prophet. Hinduism may be regarded as a henotheistic religion, meaning that it is based on the worship of a primary god, Brahman, but various other deities exist in the religion as well. Three gods, Brahma, Vishnu, and Shiva, and other deities are considered manifestations of and are worshipped as incarnations of Brahman.

Hindus believe that the purpose of existence is to realize the divine nature of life. Each life, whether it be of a man or an animal, has a soul. These souls are continually passing through stages of birth, life, death, and rebirth in a cycle called reincarnation. The purpose of reincarnation is to liberate oneself from his ego and thus be free from the pervasive suffering that it causes. The concept of karma is intrinsically bound to the principle of reincarnation in that the passage of one life to the next is determined by how the previous life was lived. Thus, performing actions that are deemed moral will allow a person to pass on to a stage that is closer to the ultimate goal of enlightenment: nirvana. During this final stage, commonly called moksha, or unification, the soul of a person is finally rejoined with Brahman.

Mrs. Krishnamurthy is admitted to the hospital for further evaluation and treatment. Her extended family is quite large and very involved. During the patient's hospitalization, numerous relatives are constantly at the bedside. Family members often approach the nurses' station to ask questions or make requests, and it is difficult for family members to restrict their time to the hospital's visitation hours. Furthermore, although the patient's son is the legal surrogate decision-maker, the family prefers to arrive at all decisions by consensus. This is a source of frustration for several of the nurses and physicians who feel that that actions of her family and their approach to decision making are preventing Mrs. Krishnamurthy from being treated appropriately or in a timely manner.

4   What are the cultural dimensions to the actions of the patient's family?

In general, U.S. culture is characterized as being more individualistic, assertive, competitive, achievement-oriented, and focused on mastery over one's environment. In contrast, traditional Asian Indian culture emphasizes strong allegiance to family, restraint of emotional expression, and a deep sense of obligation to older people. Large, extended, closely knit families are often a significant element of the Indian social tradition. Without discounting the role of acculturation, in this context, communal and familial deliberation is more prevalent among Asian Indian families, as distinct from the Western, autonomy-driven framework for decision making.

Medical culture often frames the interaction as one-to-one versus one-to-group, as in family. The majority of patients are group-oriented in terms of families or communities. Learning about decision making within family systems is essential for effective and efficient communication. Caregivers conditioned to the approach where decisions are ultimately made by a single responsible individual may find it difficult to engage families where decisions reflect familial consensus and agreement. These difficult situations require respect, patience, efforts at understanding families' cultural values, timely discussions focused on the best interest of the patient, and the negotiation of limits and boundaries. In large families, identifying an appropriate individual to be the point of contact between the care team and the family can be very helpful.

> In addition, there are other sources of conflict around her care. Mrs. Krishnamurthy is less comfortable with male nurses assisting in the personal aspects of her daily care. Also, she declines to eat the hospital food, despite a normal swallowing evaluation, and her food intake is minimal for several days. Her family begins to bring Indian meals prepared at home, which she eats avidly. This soon becomes a point of conflict with the family as the care team feels that she should be adhering to a low-sodium diet to assist in controlling her blood pressure.

5   In what way might cultural issues related to gender lead to conflict in the clinical setting?

Indian culture and traditions regarding personal space and touching differ from those of Western cultures. Physical interactions across gender lines are more restricted, which may become an issue in a clinical setting. This can be negotiated with patients as much as possible, depending on the clinical setting and the availability of the care they request. The patient can be told that the team will try to accommodate his/her requests as much as possible but cannot always do so, and that the first goal is to provide good care to the patient.

6   How do the dietary preferences of this patient impact her care?

Indian diet and cuisine differ substantially from Western foods, and patients may not find hospital food very palatable. This can impact the hospital experience of inpatients who find it very difficult to adjust to new foods, and therefore, it is more likely that food would be brought in by the patient's family. This may or may not be compatible with medical considerations, depending on the patient's diagnosis. It would be reasonable in the management of this patient to consult a registered dietitian (RD) who could advise the family on culturally appropriate meals that would still be healthy. Patients who have had a stroke may benefit from a low-salt diet and need culturally appropriate recipes and guidance, which a nutritionist can offer. Blended spices, such as those found in curry, may contain salt, but may not be recognized as a source of salt by the family.

> *Mrs. Krishnamurthy is seen in the neurology clinic 2 months after her discharge. Her daughter-in-law accompanies her and interprets for her, although she is not as facile with English as her husband. The daughter-in-law wonders if her cognitive function has been worsening since her recent discharge from the hospital. Mrs. Krishnamurthy is now able to do very little for herself independently other than dress and feed herself, and she needs help bathing. She is also more socially withdrawn. When asked if she has tried anything that seems to help her, the patient's daughter-in-law volunteers that, on a relative's recommendation, she is seeing an Ayurvedic medicine practitioner and has undergone a number of detoxifying therapies. Mrs. Krishnamurthy is also taking a combination of herbal remedies and maintains a diet that balances certain flavors, temperatures, and consistencies of food. She does not know to what degree this has been helping her mother-in-law.*

7 How do culturally related alternative medical treatments affect her "Western" medical care?

In general, it is important to appreciate that many cultures also have belief systems regarding health, healing, and medical treatment. Although these nonallopathic therapies may seem foreign or without scientific merit, it is important to respectfully, and in a nonjudgmental way, ask about their usage by the patient. In India, for example, Ayurvedic medicine is a very common practice. This therapy constitutes a comprehensive system of medical practice based on fundamentally different principles from that of Western medicine and relies on very different diagnostic and therapeutic approaches. This form of medicine focuses on reestablishing the harmony between mind, body, and nature through yoga, diet, herbs, intestinal cleansing, massage, and aromatherapy. Instruction for treatment is derived from the ancient Hindu text *Atharva Veda*. Ayurveda rests upon the *prana*, a fundamental energy that enlivens body and mind. The *prana* is made up of five elements: ether, fire, water, air, and earth. These elements are subdivided into *doshas*, unique patterns of qualities that make up an individual's *praktiti*, or essence. Illness occurs due to an imbalance in a person's essence or environment. Stress, frustration, environment, and diet all contribute to this imbalance. Each patient receives a specialized treatment of exercise, eating, sleeping, and procedures based on the imbalances of his/her *doshas*.

  Patients should not have to sacrifice all other treatment options in order to receive Western medical therapies. Rather, health care professionals should seek ways to safely complement allopathic treatments with alternative and/or nonconventional approaches.

> *Since Mrs. Krishnamurthy's discharge from the hospital, other extended family members have been watching her and the grandchildren during the day. Her daughter-in-law suspects that she should not be left alone unsupervised. The daughter-in-law is distressed by the growing demands of her mother-in-law's condition, which is imposing on her time and career goals. Although the family's income was sufficient to support either a nursing facility or a home health aid, the family is reluctant to extend the duty for caring for the patient beyond the bounds of the family. After careful consideration, the daughter-in-law decided to forego a postdoctoral position for the time being in order to care for her children and mother-in-law.*

8 What cultural issues impact decisions regarding long-term care for this patient?

Caring for a family member with physical or cognitive impairments can result in both physical and mental stress for the caregivers. Further, family members who provide care for a cognitively impaired elder can experience social isolation and loneliness due to the elder's inability to engage in conversation, return or express affection, and/or participate in social activities. Although social changes have made it more acceptable, the decision to place a loved one in a nursing home can still be difficult. This decision may be especially difficult for families whose cultural values strongly obligate them to personally care for the elderly relative. For many families, including Asian Indian, these obligations can be very compelling and may make them less likely to relinquish their elders to the care of another person or a nursing home, despite the financial ability to support such a transition.

> *Two years later, Mrs. Krishnamurthy suffers another stroke that leaves her with significant neurological deficits. Now completely unable to care for herself, Mrs. Krishnamurthy requires 24-hour care, which includes*

assistance with dressing and eating. At this point, the family decides that they can no longer take care of her alone. They reluctantly hire a caretaker to be with her at home during the day. At this stage, her physicians recognize that questions about end-of-life decision making have become pertinent. Although the son was legally empowered to make these decisions, the issue was discussed at a large family gathering. After much discussion, it is decided that Mrs. Krishnamurthy would not want to prolong her life by extraordinary medical measures. One component of this decision has to do with her spiritual beliefs. She is a firm believer in reincarnation.

9   What cultural and religious issues relate to decisions about end-of-life care for this patient?

Ideally, well before catastrophic or end-of-life events, physicians should inquire about advanced directives. Unquestionably, ethnic and/or religious values may loom large at the end-of-life. They may inform decisions about end-of-life care; guide the process by which decisions are made; influence willingness or reluctance to accept pain management or palliative treatment; and determine the rituals of death. Although respect and support of the family is of great importance, the goal should always be to ensure that decisions and treatments are consistent with the goals and values of the patient. If the clinician is unfamiliar with the values and practices of a patient's culture, it is both appropriate and helpful to ask the family about their understanding of death and the rituals of death that are important to them. This is also a situation in which pastoral care may be helpful. Evaluating the degree of adherence, beliefs, and practices is imperative to respectfully support patients at their time of death.

In terms of end-of-life and death, many Asian Indian Hindu patients may prefer to die at home, and some will want to return to India to one of the sacred cities for their death. The notion that suffering is inevitable and the result of karma may lead to reluctance to accept medications for pain control. Family members are likely to gather in large numbers as death approaches. Chanting, prayer, the burning of incense, and other rituals are very common. Once the patient has died, ideally the family should be the only ones to touch the body, and thus the hospital staff should touch the patient after death as little as possible. Traditionally, observant Hindus have a family member of the same sex clean the body, wrapping it in a red cloth after it has been cleaned. Preference is typically for cremation.

End-of-Life Decisions

Technological and medical advancements have significantly improved the ability to keep permanently unconscious or terminally ill patients alive through artificial means. As long as the patient is mentally competent, he or she has ultimate authority over such decisions. When the patient loses the ability to communicate or make judgments, the situation becomes more complicated. With such advancement also come the questions of end-of-life decisions.

Such decisions are never clear-cut and are oftentimes debated among family, friends, and health professionals. Some believe that artificial treatments may eventually restore the patient to acceptable qualities of life, whereas others view them as unnecessarily prolonging the dying process. As of now, the best way for a patient to express his or her wishes during this difficult time is to make prior preparations in the form of advance directives. An advance directive can be a living will, a document through which the patient directs the doctor to withdraw or continue lifesaving interventions, and/or a medical directive, which allows the patient to name a trusted individual to make end-of-life decisions.

References: Case 10

British Broadcasting Company. Religion and Ethics: Hinduism. Available at: http://bbc.co.uk/religion/religions/hindusim/intro2.shtml.

Firth S. End-of-life: a Hindu view. *Lancet* 2005;366:682–6.

Lan P. Subcontracting filial piety. Elder care in ethnic Chinese immigrant families in California. *J Fam Issues* 2002;7:812–35.

Jayaram V. (2006). Hinduism: main beliefs. Available at: http://hinduwebsite.com/beliefs.asp.

Kalavar J.M., Van Willigen J. Older Asian Indians resettled in America: narratives about households, culture and generation. *J Cross Cult Gerontol* 2005;20:213–30.

Ontario Consultants on Religious Tolerance: Hinduism. Available at: http://www.religioustolerance.org/hinduism.htm.

Schur D., Whitlatch C.J. Circumstances leading to placement: a difficult care giving decision. *Lippincott Case Manag* 2003;8:187–95.

Sharma H., Chandola H.M., Singh G., Basisht G. Utilization of Ayurveda in healthcare: an approach for prevention, health promotion, and treatment of disease. Part 1: Ayurveda, the science of life. *J Altern Complement Med* 2007;13(9):1011–9.

Sharma H., Chandola H.M., Singh G., Basisht G. Utilization of Ayurveda in healthcare: an approach for prevention, health promotion, and treatment of disease. Part 2: Ayurveda in primary healthcare. *J Altern Complement Med* 2007;13:1135–50.

Whitlatch C.J., Schur D., Noelker L.S., Ejaz F.K., Looman W.J. The stress process of family caregiving in institutional settings. *Gerontologist* 2001;41:462–73.

CASE 11

Carlos Cruz

A 34-year-old Mexican man with sleep apnea and metabolic syndrome

Indira Gurubhagavatula, MD,[1] Lisa Hark, PhD, RD,[2] and Sharon L. Drozdowsky, MES[3]

[1]University of Pennsylvania School of Medicine, Veterans Affairs Medical Center of Philadelphia, PA, USA
[2]Jefferson Medical College, Philadelphia, PA, USA
[3]Washington State Department of Labor and Industries, Tumwater, WA, USA

Educational Objectives

- Discuss how to effectively use a medical interpreter.
- Relate the importance of eliciting the patient's explanatory model.
- Define how sociocultural factors may influence the health care decisions of patients.

TACCT Domains: 4, 5

Case Summary, Questions and Answers

Mr. Carlos Cruz is a 34-year-old Mexican immigrant who went to the Emergency Department (ED) because of several days of upper respiratory tract symptoms. A chest x-ray revealed a small lung nodule of unknown significance. He was felt to have a viral syndrome and was given an appointment to follow-up in the pulmonary clinic in 10 days for further evaluation of the nodule. After missing his initial and two rescheduled appointments in the pulmonary clinic, one of the clinic nurses calls

---

Achieving Cultural Competency: A case-based approach to training health professionals, 1st edition. Edited by L Hark, H DeLisser. © 2009 Blackwell Publishing, ISBN: 9781405180726.

his home to encourage him to keep his appointment scheduled for next week. As she speaks with him, she is not confident that her message is understood.

1 Given the nurse's concerns about poor communication, what is the appropriate next step for this patient?

The essential point is that the nurse (or any other health care provider who believes that there is a language barrier) needs to follow through on her concern. In the immediate situation, she has two options. She could have one of her bilingual staff join the conversation (probably the better option), or she could ask the patient if there is someone else at home with him who is more proficient in English who could come to the phone either now or at a later time. By saying, *"Mr. Cruz, I am not sure I explained everything well enough for you to understand,"* the nurse is able to address her concerns without causing embarrassment for the patient or making him defensive. Subsequently, the office staff needs to be informed so that they can ensure that a trained interpreter either live or via phone will be present at the time of Mr. Cruz's visit. Information regarding the proper positioning of an interpreter are described in Appendix 1.

After completing the call, the nurse discusses the patient with Dr. Ross, one of the staff physicians, and expresses frustration over communicating with patients who can't speak English. She states, "These people never keep their appointments. I don't know why we waste our time tracking them down."

2 How should Dr. Ross respond?

Before responding, it is important to understand what the nurse is saying and why she is saying it. Although her comments may reflect her stress level, her statement could also reflect a bias toward ethnic immigrants. For Dr. Ross, this is an opportunity to initiate a conversation that acknowledges the primary importance of compassion toward patients and the possibility that cultural and ethnic factors may play a role in patient behavior. Further, there may well be other issues, specific and unique to this patient, which may be contributing to his failure to keep appointments. For example, Mr. Cruz may not feel comfortable disclosing his immigration status if he is an undocumented/illegal immigrant. In addition, his work schedule or other medical conditions may have been interfered with his ability to keep his appointments.

> *A week later, Mr. Cruz is in fact present at the clinic for his initial visit. When called by the nurse, he is sound asleep and snoring loudly in the waiting room. She wakes him up with difficulty and takes him to the exam room, where an interpreter is present. With the interpreter's help, Dr. Ross ascertains that Mr. Cruz is a truck driver and has an irregular work schedule that caused him to miss his appointments because he is either on the road or sleeping after work. Upon further questioning, it is clear that Mr. Cruz has multiple symptoms of sleep apnea and he is impaired by daytime sleepiness. Dr. Ross orders an expedited sleep study that confirms a diagnosis of severe sleep apnea, and he is prescribed continuous positive airway pressure (CPAP) therapy. He is instructed to use the CPAP machine during all periods of sleep in order to minimize his risk of falling asleep while driving. He is told that his usage of the CPAP will be monitored through a small electronic chip in the CPAP device. He is further informed that if he does not comply, and if he is still sleepy while driving, Dr. Ross is obligated under state law to report him to the Department of Transportation for possible suspension of his commercial driver's license. He is advised to make sure he sleeps for 7.5 to 8 hours each night with the CPAP machine on, to limit alcohol and sedating medications, and is educated about safe driving habits. He is told to return to the clinic in 1 month.*

3   How should Dr. Ross go about determining whether Mr. Cruz understands his diagnosis of sleep apnea and its treatment?

Ensuring that a patient understands his/her diagnosis is critical to promoting adherence (compliance) to recommended or prescribed treatments. One important element of accomplishing this is eliciting the patient's explanatory model of illness, which is described in detail in Appendix 2. As noted by Carrillo, "A patient enters the physician's office with certain beliefs, concerns, and expectations about his or her illness and the medical encounter. This conceptualization of the illness experience can be described as the patient's explanatory model. This is the patient's understanding of the cause, severity, and prognosis of an illness; the expected treatment; and how the illness affects his or her life. In essence, it is the meaning of the illness for the patient. Patient's explanatory models of illness are to a large extent culturally determined ... "

Sleep Apnea and Ethnic Minorities

A number of recent studies have shown a similar prevalence of obstructive sleep apnea in individuals from different ethnic groups. However, the importance of established risk factors for obstructive sleep apnea appears to vary between ethnic groups. A higher prevalence of obesity is related to an increased prevalence of obstructive sleep apnea among Native Americans and Hispanics. In contrast, obstructive sleep apnea in Asian populations tends to be associated with craniofacial structure peculiarities rather than obesity. Compared with Caucasians, African Americans experience a higher prevalence of apnea, which tends to be more severe and affects individuals of younger age groups. An increased severity of obstructive sleep apnea among elderly African Americans compared with Caucasians has been reported.

Mr. Cruz returns in 1 month, and his symptoms are minimally improved. The CPAP usage is checked and indicates that he has used it only 20% of the time and for less than 4 hours each night.

4   How should Dr. Ross address the patient's low CPAP adherence?

Most patients with severe sleep apnea, particularly those who are very sleepy, feel significantly better when they use the CPAP device as recommended. They notice significant improvements in daytime sleepiness and, as a result, tend to use CPAP more consistently. It is therefore worrisome, given the severity of Mr. Cruz's apnea, that he is still not using the CPAP device. This strongly suggests there are other factors that may be compromising his adherence. As a truck driver, Mr. Cruz's poor adherence also has broader implications with respect to occupational safety.

It would be important to begin by again ensuring that Mr. Cruz understands his disease and its treatment. Assuming he understands how to use the CPAP machine, the next step would be to ascertain the barriers he encountered when using this device. Given that his low adherence may potentially involve embarrassing, sensitive, and/or personal issues, it is important to continue this conversation with nonjudgmental, open-ended questions.

It is essential to separate patient-related factors (social stigma of CPAP, stigma of diagnosis, health and cultural belief system that promotes or dissuades compliance) from machine-related factors (the CPAP machine is too noisy, the mask is leaking, the mask irritates the skin, the pressure is uncomfortable). Patients may worry about how the CPAP device will impact their social functioning, including their sexual behavior. Since 80% of patients with sleep apnea are obese, their self-esteem may also be low, which could affect their motivation to adhere to the treatment. For this patient, given that he is a truck driver, barriers that may have influenced his adherence include sleeping in his truck on a regular basis and being on the road most of the time.

Occupational Safety

The association between sleep apnea and sleepiness should be highlighted in the population of commercial drivers. This is because sleepiness among commercial drivers impairs task performance and accounts for 31% to 41% of major crashes of commercial vehicles. Overall, large trucks are involved in nearly a half-million traffic accidents each year. These accidents injure 130,000 victims each year and incur huge costs. Although we know little about the role of obstructive sleep apnea in crashes in commercial vehicles, we do know that drivers of passenger cars who have obstructive sleep apnea experience increased crash risk. A recent meta-analysis quantified a 2.5-fold increase in crash-risk among sleep apnea sufferers.

5 Now that communication issues have been discussed, what specific dietary recommendations would be appropriate and realistic for Mr. Cruz to implement?

Mr. Cruz's labs and physical exam revealed elevated triglycerides and blood sugar, low HDL-C, borderline hypertension, and an abnormally high waist circumference. He therefore meets all five of the criteria for the diagnosis of metabolic syndrome (MES). He is at risk for developing diabetes and hypertension. Mr. Cruz's current diet is high in total fat, saturated fat, cholesterol, sodium, and sugar.

He is also obese, with a BMI of 32 and a waist circumference of 43 inches. At present, there is no single diet recommended for all individuals with Metabolic Syndrome therefore, it is best to focus on the specific patient's metabolic alterations when offering dietary advice.

Mr. Cruz's current job is very stressful; he is frequently on the road; he does not have time to exercise; and he has limited choices for healthy foods. Obviously these are all challenges for Mr. Cruz to improve his health. Because of his family history of obesity, diabetes, and hypertension, he is at risk of also developing these medical problems. It is important to help him understand that his current diet may make it more likely that he will develop those conditions. His goals should therefore include reducing his total calories, fat, saturated fat, sodium, sugar, cholesterol, and alcohol intake. Nutrition should also be encouraged from the standpoint of Mr. Cruz refueling his body just as he refuels his truck. Good eating practices will allow his body to perform at its best and provide extra energy and increased alertness for his long hours on the road.

To improve dietary adherence, Mr. Cruz should be advised to include more fruits and vegetables in his diet. This approach will increase fiber intake and reduce constipation, a frequent complaint of truck drivers. Examples of healthy snacks and tips for eating on the road are included in Tables 11.1 and 11.2.

6 How can Mr. Cruz increase his physical activity level?

The Institute of Medicine recommends 1 hour of physical activity daily for health maintenance. The American Heart Association calls

Table 11.1 Healthy snacks for the road

Bananas	Low-salt tomato juice	
100% juice	Baby carrots	Apples
Raisins	Celery	Oranges
Pretzels	Snap peas	Pears
Fig cookies	Grape or cherry tomatoes	Plums
Graham crackers	Grapes	Broccoli
Whole-grain crackers	Cherries	Other fresh produce

Source: Sharon Drozdowsky, Division of Occupational Safety and Health, Washington State Department of Labor and Industries, 2009. Used with permission.

Table 11.2 Tips for eating on the road

- It's all about choice as well as portions.
  - ○ Ask for nutritional information at the places you like to eat.
  - ○ Ask "What do I like and what do I need?" vs. "What do I want?"
- Have a plan.
  - ○ Walk in knowing what you will choose based on what you need.
  - ○ Stick to your plan.
- Request that food is prepared the way you want it, e.g. no gravy, broiled rather than fried, dressing on the side for you to control.
- Look for steamed, baked, broiled, braised, poached, or grilled and skip the sautéed, pan-fried, or deep-fried items.
- Look for health-focused entrees.
- Visualize the plate as a box of crayons. Keep in mind that a colorful plate containing more veggies than meat should be a goal!
- Forget the "clean plate" notion. At restaurants, ask for a doggie bag and then refrigerate it for your next meal.
- **Don't** ask for *super-size* or *value-size* items.

Source: Sharon Drozdowsky, Division of Occupational Safety and Health, Washington State Department of Labor and Industries, 2009. Used with permission.

on health professionals to prescribe 30 minutes or more of brisk walking on most or all days of the week. The greatest health benefits from an increase in physical activity occur when sedentary individuals incorporate moderate-intensity exercise as part of their lifestyle. Low-intensity exercise can have a significant impact, and it may be easier to get patients to comply with less intensive exercise regimens. Compliance declines as frequency increases. Encourage patients to find their own comfort level when it comes to physical activity. The goal for clinicians is to help each patient find a level of activity that they can accomplish over the long term. A combination of resistance and aerobic exercise is advisable, but any activity is better than none; patients who have been sedentary need to start with walking and increase duration and intensity gradually.

Mr. Cruz should exercise 30 to 60 minutes per day, on most days. Point out that exercise will make him healthier, reduce stress, help with sound sleep, improve his self-esteem, and make moving easier. Exercise will help muscles and joints become stronger, and a strong

Table 11.3 Tips for exercising on the road

- Walk at rest stops and truck stops (around facility or on walking path nearby).
- Walk around truck or bus several times at each stop.
- Walk when truck is being loaded/unloaded at the delivery site.
- Park far from the building.
- Take portable exercise equipment (such as stretch bands) in the truck.
- Ride a stationary bike at a truck stop fitness center.
- Jump rope in the rest stop parking lot.
- Pack low-weight dumbbells or cans to do arm curls.
- Use resistant elastic bands for 5–10 minutes at rest stops.
- Do crunches or push-ups in your cab (build up to this).
- Tighten stomach muscles while driving, hold for 30 seconds, then release.

Source: Sharon Drozdowsky, Division of Occupational Safety and Health, Washington State Department of Labor and Industries, 2009. Used with permission.

body is less susceptible to strains, sprains, and other injuries. Ways to exercise on the road are shown in Table 11.3.

References: Case 11

Ancoli-Israel S., Klauber M.R., Stepnowsky C., Estline E., Chinn A., Fell R. Sleep-disordered breathing in African-American elderly. *Am J Respir Crit Care Med* 1995;152:1946–9.

Aranguri C., Davidson B., Ramirez R. Patterns of communication through interpreters: a detailed sociolinguistic analysis. *J Gen Intern Med* 2006;21:623–9.

Becker H.F., Jerrentrup A., Ploch T., et al. Effect of nasal continuous positive airway pressure treatment on blood pressure in patients with obstructive sleep apnea. *Circulation* 2003;107(1):68–73.

Boule, N.A., Haddad E., Kenny, G.P., et al. Effect of exercise or glycemic control and BMI in type 2 diabetes: a meta-analysis of controlled clinical trials. *JAMA* 2001;286:1218–27.

Carrillo J.E., Green A.R., Betancourt J.R. Cross-cultural primary care: a patient-based approach. *Ann Intern Med* 1999;130:829–34.

Chen A. Doctoring across the language divide. *Health Aff* 2006;25:808–13.

Dietary Reference Intakes For Energy, Carbohydrates, Fiber, Fat, Fatty Acids, Cholesterial, Protein and Amino Acids. Institute of Medicine, National Academies Press, Washington DC, 2002.

Dysart-Gale D. Communication, models, professionalism, and the work of medical interpreters. *Health Commun* 2005;17:91–103.

Flores G. The impact of medical interpreter services on the quality of health-care: a systematic review. *Med Care Res Rev* 2005;62:255–99.

George C.F. Reduction in motor vehicle collisions following treatment of sleep apnoea with nasal CPAP. *Thorax* 2001;56(7):508–12.

Harsch I.A., Schahin S.P., Radespiel-Troger M., et al. Continuous positive airway pressure treatment rapidly improves insulin sensitivity in patients with obstructive sleep apnea syndrome. *Am J Respir Crit Care Med* 2004; 169(2):156–62.

Hla K.M., Skatrud J.B., Finn L., et al. The effect of correction of sleep-disordered breathing on BP in untreated hypertension. *Chest* 2002;122(4): 1125–32.

Howard M.E., Desai A.V., Grunstein R.R., et al. Sleepiness, sleep disordered breathing and accident risk factors in commercial vehicle drivers. *Am J Respir Crit Care Med* 2004;170:1014.

Hsieh E. Conflicts in how interpreters manage their roles in provider-patient interactions. *Soc Sci Med* 2006;62:721–30.

Hsieh E. Understanding medical interpreters: reconceptualizing bilingual health communication. *Health Commun* 2006;20:177–86.

Ip M.S., Lam B., Ng M.M., et al. Obstructive sleep apnea is independently associated with insulin resistance. *Am J Respir Crit Care Med* 2002;165(5):670–6.

Ip M.S., Lam B., Tang L.C., Lauder I.J., Ip T.Y., Lam W.K. A community study of sleep-disordered breathing in middle-aged Chinese women in Hong Kong: prevalence and gender differences. *Chest* 2002;125:127–34.

Kim J., In K., Kim J. Prevalence of sleep-disordered breathing in middle-aged Korean men and women. *Am J Respir Crit Care Med* 2004;170:1108–13.

Kleinman A., Eisenberg L., Good B. Culture, illness, and care: clinical lessons from anthropological and cross-cultural research. *Ann Intern Med* 1978; 88:251–88.

Lin H.S., Zuliani G., Amjad E.H., et al. Treatment compliance in patients lost to follow-up after polysomnography. *Otolaryngol Head Neck Surg* 2007; 136:236–40.

Marin J.M. Long-term cardiovascular outcomes in men with obstructive sleep apnoea-hypopnoea with or without treatment with continuous positive airway pressure: an observational study. *Lancet* 2005;365(9464):1046–53.

Peppard P.E. Prospective study of the association between sleep-disordered breathing and hypertension. *N Engl J Med* 2000;342(19):1378–84.

Pepperell J.C. Ambulatory blood pressure after therapeutic and subtherapeutic nasal continuous positive airway pressure for obstructive sleep apnoea: a randomised parallel trial. *Lancet* 2002;359(9302):204–10.

Punjabi N.M. Sleep-disordered breathing and insulin resistance in middle-aged and overweight men. *Am J Respir Crit Care Med* 2002;165(5):677–82.

Redline S., Tishler P.V., Hans M.G., Tosteson T.D., Strohl K.P., Spry K. Racial differences in sleep-disordered breathing in African-Americans and caucasians. *Am J Respir Crit Care Med* 1997;155:186–92.

Romero C.M. Using medical interpreters. *Am Fam Physician* 2004;69:2720–2.

Sassani A. Reducing motor-vehicle collisions, costs, and fatalities by treating obstructive sleep apnea syndrome. *Sleep* 2004;27(3):453–8.

Shahar E. Sleep-disordered breathing and cardiovascular disease: cross-sectional results of the Sleep Heart Health Study. *Am J Respir Crit Care Med* 2001;163(1):19–25.

Sleep apnea, sleepiness and driving risk. *Am J Respir Crit Care Med* 1994;150:1463–73.

Stoohs R.A. Sleep and sleep-disordered breathing in commercial long-haul truck drivers. *Chest* 1995;107(5):1275–82.

Strohl K.P., Redline S. Recognition of obstructive sleep apnea. *Am J Respir Crit Care Med* 1996;154(2 Pt 1):279–89.

Teran-Santos J., Jimenez-Gomez A., Cordero-Guevara J. The association between sleep apnea and the risk of traffic accidents. *N Engl J Med* 1999;340(11):847–51.

Udwadia Z.F., Doshi A.V., Lonkar S.G., Singh C.I. Prevalence of sleep-disordered breathing and sleep apnea in middle-aged urban Indian men. *Am J Respir Crit Care Med* 2004;169:168–73.

Weaver T.E. Adherence to positive airway pressure therapy. *Curr Opin Pulm Med* 2006;12:409–13.

Young T. The occurrence of sleep-disordered breathing among middle-aged adults. *N Engl J Med* 1993;328:1230–5.

Young T. Sleep-disordered breathing and motor vehicle accidents in a population-based sample of employed adults. *Sleep* 1997;20:608–13.

Young T., Shahar E., Nieto F.J. Predictors of sleep-disordered breathing in community-dwelling adults: the Sleep Heart Health Study. *Arch Intern Med* 2002;162:893–900.

CASE 12

Denise Smith

A 41-year-old Caucasian woman with asthma

John Paul Sánchez MD, MPH,[1] *Nelson Felix Sánchez, MD,*[2] *and Ana Núñez, MD*[3]

[1] Jacobi Medical Center, Albert Einstein College of Medicine, Bronx, NY, USA
[2] Memorial Sloan-Kettering Cancer Center, New York, NY, USA
[3] Drexel University College of Medicine, Philadelphia, PA, USA

Educational Objectives

- Explain the relevance of sexual orientation when addressing behavior modification.
- Describe how an individual's desired role in the community influences behavior.
- Examine different family structures and the influence of family members on an individual's behavior.
- Discuss how culturally tailored programming can facilitate behavior modification, such as smoking cessation, among marginalized groups.

TACCT Domains: 1, 2, 4, 6

Case Summary, Questions and Answers

Denise Smith is a 41-year-old Caucasian woman who has lived in New York City her entire life. For the past 10 years she has shared an apartment with another woman who has two children, ages 11 and 13 years. She works as a security guard at a local school but is also a

Achieving Cultural Competency: A case-based approach to training health professionals,
1st edition. Edited by L Hark, H DeLisser. © 2009 Blackwell Publishing,
ISBN: 9781405180726.

well-known party promoter and event planner in her community. Until her recent employment as a security guard, she did not have health insurance and her only contact with the health care system in the past 5 years consisted of four visits to the Emergency Department (ED) for shortness of breath and wheezing.

Over the past 5 days she has had a viral syndrome, accompanied by a nonproductive cough and worsening shortness of breath. She visits the local health department clinic (her last visit was 7 years ago) for a refill of her asthma inhaler.

As she enters the waiting room, she draws stares from other patients and staff. She has a very short, dark haircut and is wearing black sunglasses, black slacks, a white button-down shirt, and baggy blazer. She walks up to the front desk to check in for her appointment and the clerk responds, "Sir, please write your name down and you'll be called shortly." A half hour later, a nurse calls out, "Denise Smith, please come to the door." On coming to the door, the nurse says to Ms. Smith, "Sir, I was calling for your wife." There are several snickers from other patients in the waiting room.

Ms. Smith pushes open the door and walks through. She refuses to allow the nurse to take any vitals and asks to see the doctor immediately. The nurse hands the patient chart to the doctor and informs him that the patient is in the room. On entering the room, the doctor asks, "Sir, has your wife stepped out to the bathroom?" Disgusted by the confusion once again, Ms. Smith angrily responds, "No, I'm Denise. Doesn't anyone know who I am? Look, I've been waiting here for an hour and all I need is a refill for my asthma pump. Can't you just do that for me?"

1 What are the issues surrounding the misidentification of this patient?

This case illustrates the tendency to interpret human identification from the context of "what are you?" rather than "who are you?" Ms. Smith's interaction also affords an opportunity to examine the multiple influences of gender and identity on her health status. First, the front desk staff did not notice her name as she signed in. Second, the staff rebuked her attempt to enter the clinic when her name was called. She then feels insulted as she enters the examination room; most people, when mistaken for a gender other than their own, do feel insulted. Ironically, most lesbian patients are invisible to their physician and have been named the "invisible minority." They appear like any other women in the practice and their reticence to divulge "personal information" is misread as shyness, lack of trust, or merely being too busy to answer the questions.

Why did the staff misidentify her? Many people are raised to expect sexual stereotypes. For example, "girls wear pink" and "boys wear blue," and only boys have shaved heads and only girls have pierced ears. Androgynistic (not having characteristics, dress, appearance, or behavior that are distinguishably masculine or feminine) appearing people may confuse service professionals, such as front desk, clinic staff, or physicians. The majority of people in the U.S. assume that all people are heterosexual. The reflex questions, "Are you married (implied being to a man)?" and "What is your husband's name? provide two common examples of presumed heterosexism. As in most errors in medicine, cutting corners and working rapidly can also result in adverse outcomes.

From a communication perspective, adopting an approach of asking, rather than assuming, is essential to avoiding unintentional insults or conveying an inclusive office setting for all patients. In this case, the front desk clerk, the nurse, and the doctor mistakenly identified Ms. Smith as a man rather than a woman, based on her attire. Aside from appearance, paying attention to how a patient introduces herself (i.e., Ms. Denise Smith), what gender is checked off on the intake or registration form, or what name appears on the insurance card helps to better clarify how the patient wishes to be identified. The health professionals could have rephrased their questions to be more culturally sensitive. The front desk clerk could have simply stated, "Please write your name down." The nurse could have stated, "Hi, I'm Nurse Williams. And you are?" And the doctor could have stated, "Hi, I'm Dr. Jones. Are you Denise Smith?"

2   What are the implications of misidentification on development of rapport with a patient and a perceived sense of safety in a health care setting?

It is unlikely that a patient will feel safe if he or she is in an environment where "they don't even know who you are." There are ample messages by the media of patient misidentification, error, and harm as a result of medical misadventures. It is easy to forget that, in the environment where physicians feel comfortable with the routines and setting, most patients are still extraordinarily anxious even when they are healthy, much less if they are sick and feel ill.

Ms. Smith, in this case, is a woman who is a lesbian, but she could also have been a heterosexual artist or an avid sports enthusiast. In medicine, we often use our eyes to decide and define what (and who) we see. This proclivity fails us, more often than not. We need to ask, facilitate the discussion, and hear who the person defines herself as, rather than making judgments based on an impression. Asking rather than assuming is a safe habit to prevent erroneous misattribution.

3   How should the office staff have responded to rectify this problem?

The staff members should have apologized to Ms. Smith and responded by saying, "I am so sorry, please come in. How are you today?" If they did not apologize, the issue should have been shared with the physician so that he could convey his apology for how she was treated upon arriving to the clinic.

The physician should have said "Oh, I'm so sorry; Ms. Smith, how are you? What brings you here today?" If the staff member had shared with the physician her story as in, "we called her 'a guy' by accident and she's only here for a refill of her inhaler and in a rush," he might have had advanced warning of the patient's perspectives and concerns. Working as a team and treating staff members respectfully, as well as soliciting their input on "what is going on" with a patient, are essential skills in working together and delivering unified and effective health care.

To promote an inclusive medical environment there needs to be intentional actions and trainings to raise awareness, even beyond sex role stereotypes and bias. When a lesbian patient fills out a form that has her choose married, divorced, or single, what does she select if she and her partner of 11 years can't marry in the state they live in? Does she check married and then get asked, "What does your husband do?" or does she select single and have no information about her support system or life? Intentional actions and training need to occur because good intentions are insufficient to raise insight about heterosexist assumptions as well as homophobia. Presumed heterosexism means that a person assumes everyone is heterosexual. Therefore, all women are asked if they have a boyfriend or husband; all men are asked if they have a girlfriend or a wife. By limiting options, a physician can put a patient into a position of not being truthful (telling you what you want to hear.) This is especially true if there is no preexisting relationship. Will the physician judge the patient or treat her poorly if she shares that she is a lesbian? The literature has ample examples of patients being treated harshly or poorly as a result of homophobia, so patients are not unfounded in their concern.

Because homophobia and presumed heterosexism are prevalent in mainstream culture, training sessions to discuss these issues with staff should occur and be facilitated effectively. Unless staff and clinician trainings occur, an open discussion about gay and lesbian patients cannot occur in a productive fashion. By realizing the life experience of lesbian patients and developing an empathetic perspective, all health professionals can contribute to decreasing health disparities in this population of patients.

4   What is important to understand about Ms. Smith's community?

In evaluating the sexual health of all patients, clinicians need to understand key issues about sexual orientation. Sexual orientation runs across a continuum and has three components: attraction, cognition, and behavior. Attraction or desire describes a patient's sexual affinity. Cognition is how they choose to define themselves, for example straight, bisexual, gay, or lesbian. Behavior, as it sounds, is what a patient does or doesn't do. Patients may choose to be sexually active with another person or themselves or be celibate. These three areas often cause confusion in understanding sexual behavior because they do not necessarily track together.

A woman may have sex with a man, yet identify herself as a lesbian. A woman may not have sex at all and identify herself as bisexual. A woman may be in a committed relationship with another woman but vehemently refute the label of "gay." Our patients may or may not share information with us about whom they are attracted to. They can define themselves as they see themselves: their identity. Hopefully, we can create a safe space in the medical setting to enable patients to share what they do and with whom, so that we can best serve in helping them understand their health risks.

Gay culture, like all learned behavior and cultures, has social norms, expectations, traditions, values, language (both verbal and nonverbal), and behaviors. The degree of acculturation varies from person to person, just as the role of any cultural influence is balanced by individual influence and may change over time. To make the cultural implication even more challenging, the role of being gay in a person's identity varies with age, geography, religion, ethnicity, socioeconomic status, and education. So, the role of gay culture on a patient may be one of many influences on the individual patient in front of you.

Lesbians and Health Disparities

A Lesbian is a woman who forms a primary intimate relationship with another woman and who is sexually oriented to the same sex. Estimates of the number of lesbians in the U.S. vary, but could be from 2.2 to 11.8 million people. This data range estimate applies Lauman's estimate of women who identify as lesbians (1.4%), Kinsey's' data (5-6%) and Michael's data (7.5%) on women who report same gender desire on current population (October 2007) of 153.6 million women in the U.S.

But beyond statistics, many people do not know that lesbians as a group are as diverse as any other group in the U.S. They are of all socioeconomic classes and of every ethnicity. They live in every state in the U.S. They are childless and they have children. Based on the literature, about two-thirds of them have or have had sexual intercourse with men (which influences sexual health risks.) Additionally, there are gay and lesbian staff, health professionals, and physicians who may or may not feel safe nor supported where they work.

Barriers to access health care among lesbians include: stress effects of homophobia, obesity, smoking, cardiovascular, mental health, and substance abuse issues, and cancer. Lesbian women are a difficult group to research regarding their health habits, as discrimination in the workplace as well as personal safety are issues for sexual minorities. Much of the literature about lesbian women has been collected from small numbers or from convenience samples – for example, groups of women attending a social event. The health habits of individuals who frequent social events are likely to be different than those women who do not participate in these activities or whose lives center around the raising of children. Consequently, future studies on the health of lesbians need to be designed to appropriately sample this population of women.

The doctor explains to Ms. Smith that, before he can give her any medication, he must conduct a history and physical examination. Ms. Smith agrees but urges the doctor to be quick because she's promoting an event later that evening. Her past medical history consists only of asthma, with increasing episodes of wheezing in the past 3 months, which worsen when she's chasing after kids at school and after her events in the evening. She has had the same albuterol inhaler for the past 6 months, which over the last several days she has used six to eight times each day. Over the past week, she has had a "cold" that she believes is the main cause of her worsening shortness of breath. She has a nonproductive cough but feels like there is something in her lungs. She smokes about 10 cigarettes a day, more when she's stressed, which has been the case over the past 3 months, but much less than about 5 years ago when she was smoking 1.5 packs per day. When asked if she has ever tried to quit, she avoids the question and replies, "Look I'm not here to be judged. Why does it matter if I've ever quit or how much I smoke or, for that matter, what else I do? Listen, what I do is my business. This is why I stopped coming to the doctor; all of these personal questions. The last doctor made all of these suggestions to me and my partner on how to quit and none worked. Great, now I feel more short of breath than before."

She reaches for the inhaler and takes a puff. The doctor asks to see the inhaler and discovers that it is empty. Pressed by her urgency to leave, the doctor ends the history and proceeds to the physical examination. He limits his examination to the lungs in which he hears scattered wheezing and good air entry.

"Okay, Ms. Smith, we're going to give you an asthma treatment and then I'll come back and re-assess you."

5 Why does Ms. Smith feel like she is being "judged?"

This comment may reflect anger, frustration, and hurt on a number of levels. She may be expressing residual anger over the initial encounter with the clerk, nurse, and physician. This anger was further compounded by the fact that the staff did not acknowledge their inappropriate comments either through an apology or by asking Ms. Smith her preferred terms of self-identity. This, in turn, may have led Ms. Smith to project a more "aggressive" or "hostile" demeanor that hampers effective doctor–patient communication. Ms. Smith may also be expressing frustration over a sense that, rather than addressing her asthma, the reason she came to the clinic, the doctor is focused on her smoking, a habit she has been unable to give up despite efforts to do so. In addition her comments may reflect life experiences, whether real or perceived, of bias and mistreatment in the health care system or in the wider society.

If a patient feels "judged" (i.e. dismissed, discounted, disrespected), the effectiveness of the doctor–patient interaction is jeopardized. A patient may be less willing to provide an honest or complete history of illnesses, behaviors, or existing support networks. A patient may be less inclined to undergo a more extensive or "invasive" physical examination, such as a pelvic examination, especially if they do not plan to continue care with that provider. The development and implementation of a feasible and effective treatment plan requires that the patient and physician can communicate openly about the patient's desired health outcomes, perceived obstacles, and services needed to achieve these outcomes. Developing and maintaining a strong, supportive, and comfortable relationship with patients can facilitate success throughout the doctor–patient encounter.

Thirty minutes later, the doctor returns and, on reexamination of Ms. Smiths' lungs, discovers improved air entry and no wheezing. The doctor informs Ms. Smith that her asthma was probably exacerbated by her recent cold and continued cigarette smoking. He writes prescriptions for an albuterol inhaler and 5-day course of steroids and instructs her how to assess when the inhaler is empty.

"Ms. Smith, I realize you have been unhappy with the care you have received today, and I apologize if I or my staff made you uncomfortable. If you can spare the time, I would just like to talk with you a little more about your smoking since I think it's affecting your asthma."

Ms. Smith replies, "Doctor I hear what you're saying, but I'm sure it was the cold not my smoking. I smoke every day, but my asthma only really gets bad when I also have a cold or I'm stressed. I can try and cut down, but I'm not ready to quit. Cigarettes help me relax which I need right now. I'm a party promoter, so I smoke, especially when I'm out with my girlfriends. It's a part of the scene." She explains that many of the women who attend her events at clubs and restaurants smoke.

The doctor asks, "Tell me about some of the important people in your life. I see you're wearing a ring on your wedding finger. Do you currently have a partner?"

"I have a wife."

"And do you identify with the term lesbian or another term?"

"Lesbian."

"Does your wife smoke?" "Yeah. We try not to smoke too much in the house because of our kids. Our 11 year old has asthma, and the cigarette smoke makes him cough."

Smoking Influences and Quitting Rates: Women vs. Men

In the U.S., 22% of women smoke, and there continues to be increased rates of smoking among teenage females compared with their male counterparts. The prevalence of smoking among women is positively associated with younger age, lower income, lower educational level, a disadvantaged neighborhood environment, and certain racial/ethnic groups.

Gender parity in smoking has resulted in lung cancer now being the leading cause of cancer-related deaths in women, surpassing even breast cancer.

Most smokers will require multiple attempts at quitting smoking (on average 7 to 9 sincere attempts) before they can quit, and women are no exception. Women, more often than men, however, use smoking as a weight control measure and therefore have more difficulty quitting since most ex-smokers gain weight after ceasing to smoke. Women, as compared with men, have more societal pressure about their appearance and this plays a role in their smoking-cessation challenges.

Different than men, women have much higher rates of depression with quitting. This is one of the reasons that some modalities that help mood and smoking cessation may be more useful in women. Lastly, women often benefit from culturally appropriate, social support settings to enable quitting.

6 What are some of the challenges that may make it more difficult for Ms. Smith, as a lesbian woman, to quit smoking?

Smoking rate estimates vary among lesbians from 11% to 50%. Significantly, there is evidence that lesbian women may have increased smoking rates as they age, which differs from heterosexual women, who have lower rates with aging. Lesbians have been shown to have a higher rate of anxiety and depression due to stigmatization and homophobia. Cigarette smoking may be one strategy that lesbians employ to deal with the burdens of stress and homophobia associated with their sexual orientation. Anxiety and depression can lead to isolating behaviors that further decrease social resources, and the desire to smoke often increases with anxiety and depression. It is also important to realize that some tobacco companies have demonstrated public support for lesbian, gay, bisexual, and transsexual (LGBT) organizations through financial donations and visibility at

LGBT events. This creates, in some LGBT people, a sense of loy-alty to certain brands of cigarettes. By smoking these brands, LGBT smokers believe they are supporting a company that uses advertising intended to attract LGBT consumers. Lastly, there is a paucity of research that has targeted lesbians to validate smoking cessation approaches that would be effective in this group of women.

> *Despite numerous adverse factors, Ms. Smith has attempted to quit smoking a number of times before. Ms. Smith has also successfully cut down from one to a half a pack of cigarettes per day. Her wife has also cut down, and they have seen a significant amount of monetary savings. However, despite seven prior attempts, she has been unable to quit. She has tried the nicotine patch, nicotine gum, and hypnosis. She even attended a smoking cessation support group with her wife but felt the group was not accepting of their lifestyle. They know that smoking does affect the health of their children and their health, but they are unable to quit.*

7   What can Ms. Smith do and how can the physicians help motivate her behavior change?

Assess willingness to quit. The physician needs to first determine whether Ms. Smith is, in fact, ready to quit. The literature is quite clear that, if the patient is not truly ready to make a change, sustained smoking cessation is unlikely and efforts at this time will result in patient frustration and pessimism regarding success in subsequent attempts to give up cigarettes.

Emphasize the benefits of quitting smoking. For Ms. Smith, these might include improved health and better control of her asthma; saving money (which actually can be strong a motivation for quitting); and avoiding the detrimental effects of second-hand smoke on her children, such as ear or respiratory tract infections. "Scaring" patients into quitting by simply emphasizing that smoking will kill them rarely motivates patients for long-lasting change.

Review past attempts at quitting. Her physician should acknowledge and affirm her past efforts to give up smoking and then explore what worked, even if only briefly when she previously tried to quit, and then what propelled her to "light up" again. This may be useful in highlighting her personal awareness of a more effective quitting plan.

Enlist support of loved ones. A potentially very useful strategy is to identify family members and friends who can be recruited as allies in her effort to give up cigarettes. Given that Ms. Smith's partner also smokes, it may be helpful to negotiate with her partner about setting a mutual quit day, as it is extraordinarily difficult among any couple to have one person quit while the other continues to smoke.

Develop a plan jointly with the patient. The physician can provide medical therapy for nicotine replacement and mood disturbances, referral to support groups or smoking cessation programs, including LGBT-friendly programs, and advice for dealing with withdrawal symptoms and avoiding weight gain. In developing a plan with Ms. Smith, it is essential to ask her what she can do as first steps, rather than providing numerous options of what she *should* do. The plan should include follow-up with the physician.

References: Case 12

Aaron D.J. Behavioral risk factors for disease and preventive health practices among lesbians. *Am J Public Health* 2001;91:972–5.

Bergen A.W. Cigarette smoking. *J Natl Cancer Inst* 1999;1365–75.

Census Data Facts for Features. CB08-FF.03 Jan. 2, 2008. Available at: http://www.census.gov.

Dibble S.L. Risk factors for ovarian cancer: lesbian and heterosexual women. *Oncol Nurs Forum* 2002;29:E1–7.

Dibble S., Roberts S., Nussey B. Comparing breast cancer risk between lesbians and their heterosexual sisters. *Women's Health Issues* 2004;14(2):60–8. Lesbian Health Research Center: USCF. Available at: http://www.lesbianhealthinfo.org.

Doolan D. Efficacy of smoking cessation intervention among special populations. Review of the literature from 2000 to 2005. *Nurs Res* 2006; 55(4S):S29–37.

Fagerstrom K. The epidemiology of smoking: health consequences and benefits of cessation. *Drugs* 2002;62:1–9 (suppl 2).

Fiore M.C. US public health service clinical practice guideline: treating tobacco use and dependence. *Respir Care* 2000;45(10):1200–62.

Gay and Lesbian Medical Association and LGBT Health Experts. *Healthy People 2010 Companion Document for Lesbian, Gay, Bisexual and Transgender (LGBT) Health*. Gay and Lesbian Medical Association, San Francisco, 2001.

Kaiser Permanente National Diversity Council and the Kaiser Permanente National Diversity Department. *A Provider's Handbook on Culturally Competent Care: Lesbian, Gay, Bisexual, and Transgender Populations*. Oakland, 2000.

Kinsey A.C., Pomeroy W.B., Martin, C.E., Gebhard P. *Sexual Behavior in the Human Female*. W.B. Saunders, Philadelphia, 1953.

Laumann E.O., Gagnon J.H., Michael R.T., Michaels S. *The Social Organization of Sexuality: Sexual Practices in the United States.* University of Chicago Press, Chicago, 1994.

Lehmann J.B. Development and health care needs of lesbians. *J Women's Health* 1998;7:379–87.

Michaels S. The prevalence of homosexuality in the United States. In: Cabaj R.P. & Stein T.S., eds. *Textbook of Homosexuality and Mental Health.* American Psychiatric Press, Washington DC, 1996, pp 43–63.

Mravcak S.A. Primary care for lesbians and bisexual women. *Am Fam Physician* 2006;74(2):279–86, 287–8.

Ryan H. Smoking among lesbians, gays, and bisexuals: a review of the literature. *Am J Prev Med* 2001;21:142–9.

Sanchez J.P. Cigarette smoking and lesbian and bisexual women in the Bronx. *J Community Health* 2005;30(1):23–37.

Stevens P. An analysis of tobacco industry marketing to lesbian, gay, bisexual, and transgender (LGBT) populations: strategies for mainstream tobacco and prevention. *Health Promot Pract* 2004;5(3):129S–134S.

Valanis B.G. Sexual orientation and health: comparisons in the women's health initiative sample. *Arch Fam Med* 2000;9:843.

Women and Smoking: A Report of Surgeon General. United States Public Health Service, Office of the Surgeon General, Washington DC, 2001.

CASE 13

Mae Ling Chung

A 22-year-old Chinese woman in an arranged marriage

Elizabeth Lee-Rey, MD, MPH, and Nereida Correa, MD, MPH
Albert Einstein College of Medicine, Bronx, NY, USA

Educational Objectives

- Describe the custom and marriage practices prevalent in some families within Asian communities.
- Review the issues of arranged marriage, gender roles, and their effect on the physician–patient relationship.
- Appreciate the impact of cultural influences on the choice of contraception.
- Formulate approaches to caring for this patient/couple that maximizes on establishing a sense of trust, autonomy, and independence in making health care decisions.

TACCT Domains: 1, 2, 3, 4

Case Summary, Questions and Answers

Mae Ling Chung is a 22-year-old Chinese woman who immigrated to the U.S. 2 months ago after her family arranged for her to marry Wang Chung, a 30-year-old Chinese American man who has been in the U.S. for the past 12 years. She was an elementary school piano teacher in China

---

Achieving Cultural Competency: A case-based approach to training health professionals,
1st edition. Edited by L Hark, H DeLisser. © 2009 Blackwell Publishing,
ISBN: 9781405180726.

but is currently not working. Mr. Chung had made an appointment to see a gynecologist to determine whether his wife is healthy enough to "bear" him children. Dr. Pedro Gonzalez, the physician assigned to see her, enters the room and immediately notices that Mr. Chung is sitting in one of the two chairs facing his desk, whereas Mrs. Chung is seated across the room on the examination table. When Dr. Gonzalez invites her to sit next to her husband, Mr. Chung initially resists saying, "her English is poor." Despite Dr. Gonzalez's efforts to speak to Mrs. Chung during the initial interview, Mr. Chung dominates the conversation, answering all the questions directed at Mrs. Chung except for a couple of yes/no questions. He refuses to entertain any questions related to his wife's past sexual history, indicating that these questions are irrelevant.

Arranged Marriages

An arranged marriage by definition is a marriage in which neither spouse has control over the selection of their future partner. However, both parties give full consent to the marriage. Arranged marriages have been a successful tradition of family life in many cultures for years. Although often considered by Westerners as a lost tradition of the past, arranged marriages still remain an integral facet of life in many cultures today and are an accepted practice in Iraq, Iran, Afghanistan, Africa, Japan, Indonesia, India, and Bangladesh. This also can be seen in Amish communities, appreciated in the role of Jewish matchmaker "shadchan," and evident in recent immigrants from Yemen and Albania. In China, arranged and semi-arranged marriages are still common, although the Chinese government introduced a new Marriage Law in 1980 setting the legal ages for women (20) and men (22) to marry. The law also confirmed the government's approval for free-choice marriage, right to divorce, and the elimination of child marriages. Although there are no statistics on the success rate of arranged marriages in a Western context, anecdotal evidence suggests that these relationships often fail when husbands demand total autonomy over their spouses.

1 Why might Mr. Chung be acting in this way?

His behavior could simply reflect discomfort due to an unfamiliar situation or anxiety related to his new relationship and/or his desire to have children. Another possibility is that Mrs. Chung's status as a very recent immigrant, and his sense of her limited English language proficiency, may have led Mr. Chung to see his wife as very vulnerable and in need of his protection. In addition, issues related to the arranged nature of the relationship may be at work as well. As they have been together for only a few weeks, Mr. and Mrs. Chung may not have actually discussed their past sexual histories with each other. Further, the marriage may have been agreed to based on promises of the virginity of his wife, which Mr. Chung believes to be true, and/or he does not want to hear anything that would question the notion of his wife's virginity. Mr. Chung's behavior may also reflect traditional Chinese male–female roles in the family of male dominance and female submission. And certainly, his actions may have nothing to do with any of the above. This may be who he is: a "controlling," "domineering" individual.

> Dr. Gonzalez asks Mr. Chung to leave the room so that he can examine Mrs. Chung, who up until now has not been able to say much. Mr. Chung hesitates but eventually agrees to leave, again requesting that his wife not be asked any questions related to her sexual history.

2   How might Dr. Gonzalez respond to Mr. Chung's request that questions not be asked about his wife's sexual history?

Physicians cannot agree to requests that are inconsistent with established standards of care or which are not in the best interest of the patient. Further, to promise not to ask the questions, and then do so, runs the risk of alienating Mr. Chung should he discover that the physician has lied. In this situation, the perceptive physician will realize that s/he will, however, need to take a few minutes to focus on Mr. Chung and begin the process of eliciting and understanding his goals and expectations for the care of his wife. This will aid in the development of trust and will provide information that will enable Dr. Gonzalez to negotiate a way through Mr. Chung's objections.

3   Given the behavior of Mr. Chung, what other issue should Dr. Gonzalez consider as he evaluates Mrs. Chung?

The controlling behavior of her husband should raise some concern and prompt the physician to consider and potentially screen for intimate partner violence. Although studies specific to Chinese immigrants have been limited, the available data do suggest that domestic violence is a problem in this and other Asian immigrant populations.

Although domestic violence is a problem that transcends race/ethnicity or class, there are several features of Asian communities that may increase the occurrence and/or tolerance of partner violence. These include the following:

- traditional cultural norms in which femininity is strongly associated with submissiveness;
- community denial or discounting of the problem;
- a strong emphasis on close family ties and a reluctance to do anything that would disturb the harmony or order of the family;
- fear on the part of the women of jeopardizing their immigration status;
- a lack of an extended family support in the United States;
- pressure to maintain the wider societal image of Asians as the "model minority";
- domestic relationships in which the women are financially dependent on their husbands;
- limited English proficiency;
- ignorance of (Western) legal rights and available services.

These factors, in addition to more general societal, patriarchal arrangements, cause many immigrant women to stay in abusive relationships and/or be fearful of seeking help. It is therefore essential for health care providers to the take the initiative in exploring the possibility of partner violence when it is suspected for an immigrant patient. In pursuing a suspicion of domestic violence, it is essential to do this in a way and at a time that is safe for the patient.

Indicators of an Abusive Relationship

A series of questions can be asked regarding the patient's inner thoughts and feeling or which explore the behavior of the partner to determine whether a patient's relationship with her partner may be abusive.

The Patient's Inner Thoughts and Feelings
Do you:
- feel afraid of your partner most of the time? **[This may be the most significant sign of abuse.]**
- feel emotionally numb or helpless?
- wonder if you're the one who is "crazy?"
- believe that you deserve to be mistreated or hurt?
- avoid certain topics out of fear of angering your partner?
- feel that it is impossible to do anything right for your partner?

The Partner's Belittling Behavior

Does your partner:

- humiliate, criticize, or shout at you?
- blame you for his own abusive behavior?
- ignore or put down your opinions or accomplishments?
- see you as property or a sex object, rather than as a person?
- treat you so badly that you're embarrassed for your friends or family to see you?

The Partner's Controlling Behavior

Does your partner:

- constantly check up on you?
- control where you go or what you do?
- act excessively jealous and possessive?
- prevent you from seeing your family or friends?
- limit your access to the phone, car, or money?

The Partner's Violent Threats or Behavior

Does your partner:

- have a bad and unpredictable temper?
- hurt you or threaten to hurt or kill you?
- threaten to take your children away or harm them?
- threaten to commit suicide if you leave?
- destroy your belongings?
- force you to have sex?

Adapted from: Davies P., Smith, M., de Benedictis T., Jaffe J and Segal J. Domestic violence and abuse: warning signs and symptoms of abusive relationships. Available at: http://www.helpguide.org/mental/.

As soon as Mr. Chung leaves the room, Mrs. Chung moves closer to Dr. Gonzalez, becoming more animated, smiling, and, surprisingly, speaking English well enough to be understood. She immediately thanks Dr. Gonzalez for giving her an opportunity to speak in private and tells him she is grateful to be able to use the American health care system. She explains that she only met her husband 2 months ago and that their families had arranged the marriage. Although she agreed to the arrangement and is pleased with her husband, she now feels unhappy. She begins crying and explains that she is not ready to have a baby and asks Dr. Gonzalez to prescribe "Bi Yun" (prevent pregnant) birth control. She indicates that she does not want her husband to know about her use of contraception.

4 Why might Mrs. Chung have been willing to tell Dr. Gonzalez, but not her husband, that she was not ready to have a child?

An arranged Chinese marriage is more about an obligation to one's parents than a romance and more an indication of personal self-worth and achievement for the husband. A common Chinese idiom is *"cheng jia ii ye,"* translated as "get married and start one's career." Although Mrs. Chung had accepted her marriage as an obligation to fulfill a traditional Chinese female role, now that she is in the U.S. she no longer wishes to be a dutiful "wife who hums along, while the husband sings" and is not ready to have children. From a Western perspective, steeped in the empowerment of women, this might not be seen as problematic. However, Mrs. Chung's agreement to the prearranged marriage was a commitment not only to her husband but to their respective families as well. Consistent with cultural norms, this commitment included an expectation by all involved that a child would soon follow their marriage and a family would be started. From the traditional Chinese cultural perspective, a loss of honor and subsequent disgrace results from a failure to keep one's promises. Thus, in deciding not to have a child at this time, she not only would have to face the disappointment and anger of her husband, she would have to carry the cultural burdens of breaking a promise as well as not having children (at least not immediately) and thus risk being seen as an "old virgin." Given this, and the newness of the relationship, it is not surprising that she shared her feelings with Dr. Gonzalez but not her husband.

During the visit while her husband was present, Mrs. Chung was unable to speak freely about her ambivalence regarding her prearranged role as wife and her husband's and their families' expectations for starting a family as soon as possible. She had come to see this visit as an opportunity to gain support of her desire to postpone pregnancy and was frustrated that she was unable to speak for herself while in the company of her husband. All this would not have come to the light if Dr. Gonzalez had not provided time to be alone with Mrs. Chung. This illustrates the importance of creating opportunities for patients to speak safely and not relying on family members to serve as interpreters. It also emphasizes the role that physicians can play in being advocates for vulnerable patient groups, such as immigrants with limited English proficiency.

5 Is it appropriate to prescribe contraception to this patient?

It is Mrs. Chung's right to receive all available information on her family planning options and to choose to delay pregnancy or not to become pregnant at all. However, some careful thought and consideration should go into Mrs. Chung's decision given the cultural dynamics (the immediate expectation of a child) and the nature of their relationship. The first issue is whether she will inform her husband of her intension and plans. It is not surprising, given that her marriage was arranged, that she might feel powerless or fearful to discuss this with her husband, particularly in light of his desire for a child. And such a conversation is made even more difficult by the possible dishonor and disgrace that she could bring her family if she did not have a child immediately. However, given her dependence (financial and otherwise) on her husband and her lack of familiarity with the American health care system, the best approach would be to develop a strategy of informing and including Mr. Chung in this aspect of her care. Moreover, a discussion with her husband is favored because open communication will strengthen their relationship and their marriage. If Mrs. Chung is willing to inform her husband, then Dr. Gonzalez should help her explain her perspective to Mr. Chung.

A decision to not tell her husband is Mrs. Chung's right but is fraught with risk and not likely to work in the long term. That is, her husband will likely discover that she is using contraception. Has she carefully considered his reaction should he discover that she is employing birth control without his knowledge? Would this, in turn, create issues of safety for her? Will she feel comfortable knowing that she is keeping something from her husband? These are important questions that Mrs. Chung needs to consider. If she decides not to inform her husband, then Dr. Gonzalez should reassure Mrs. Chung that he will act to preserve the confidentiality of her decision.

The second issue is the actual choice of the specific form of birth control to be employed. A complete discussion of contraception should include a description of methods, written (if she reads English) and verbal explanation of pros and cons for each method, and an opportunity for questions related to how each works. There are methods that are culturally less acceptable and/or more problematic, such as condoms and other barrier methods that require cooperation from both partners. If Mrs. Chung chooses not to disclose her use of contraception to her husband, she will need a method such as birth control pills or the Nuva Ring that is reliable but not readily noticed by her partner. However, some of these more private methods may require subsequent physician visits that may make it difficult for Mrs. Chung to conceal her contraception use from her husband.

With her husband waiting outside, the complex nature of the discussion, and Mrs. Chung's limited English proficiency, it is clear that this decision preferably should not be made after a brief or rushed conversation between the patient and the physician. There is certainly a need for a follow-up visit (in a week or two), ideally with an interpreter present, to ensure that Mrs. Chung is making an informed decision. This would also give her the opportunity to discuss the issue of birth control with her husband if she decides to inform him of her decision.

Chinese Women and Contraception

Since the inception of the Chinese government's "one-child" policy in 1979, contraception has been widely available in China. Permanent sterilization and intrauterine devices (IUDs) have been the most common forms of contraception, with historically much lower use of condoms and oral contraceptives. In the wake of increasing rates of HIV infection, the Chinese government, however, has begun to promote the use of condoms. The patterns of contraceptive use may be somewhat different in North America. In a study of 40 ethnic Chinese women in Vancouver, Canada, the methods of contraception most frequently employed were condoms ($n = 40$), rhythm method ($n = 20$), and withdrawal method ($n = 17$), typically in combination. For this group of women, only 14 have ever used oral contraceptives and only 3 had used an IUD. None had used a spermicide or an injectable contraceptive such as Depo-Provera. These data are reflective of the fact that the attitudes of ethnic Chinese women (in Canada) toward oral contraceptives are generally negative. Common concerns in this group of women are weight gain, permanent infertility, and fear of being considered promiscuous. A similar distrust of birth control pills has also been detected in ethnic Korean women (see Wiebe et al., 2002, 2004, 2006).

6   Over time, what role can Dr. Gonzalez play to help improve communication for this couple?

Dr. Gonzalez must establish a trusting rapport with Mrs. Chung in order to support and empower her to open channels of communication. He will need to establish an open, unbiased, and safe environment that will include an understanding and appreciation of individual, family, and the sociocultural and economic pressures that are impacting on this couple's ability to make family planning decisions. Mrs. Chung must struggle with becoming "the virtuous wife and good mother (*xianqi liangmu*)." She is also likely to face difficulty in obtaining the credentials needed to resume her previous career as a grade school piano teacher. Thus, if she seeks work, she may be forced to accept some form of unskilled employment (e.g. housekeeping or restaurant work). With employment opportunities often being limited and low-paying, many immigrants will have to work long hours and/or have several (part-time) jobs. And when she does have a child, child care may become a particular challenge, given its cost and the lack of support from extended family members, such as grandparents (which she would have back in China). Therefore, discussion over time of issues such as the role of honor, family obligations, work-related frustrations, and acculturation versus individual needs and expectations will be the kind of conversations that will help to establish and strengthen cross-cultural communication. Dr. Gonzalez should not feel that he can or should do this alone, but he should offer Mrs. Chung referrals to a social worker, culturally appropriate support groups, and other support systems.

Respecting and valuing Mrs. Chung's individuality will enable Dr. Gonzalez to see her needs from the most basic, such as nutrition and sustenance, to the more complex, such as self-actualization. One way of conceptualizing this is through Maslow's Hierarchy of needs, of which there are five levels that must be fulfilled in order to live a full life and feel happy. Although some of these needs are not absolutely essential, the foundations of Maslow's pyramid are indispensible, and as one moves toward the apex, more complex needs come into play. Understanding her needs for safety, security, belonging, and self-esteem will help Mrs. Chung as she transitions in this stage of her life.

Another option that is not always appropriate, but which may make sense in this situation, is for Dr. Gonzalez to suggest that he also see Mr. Chung for his health care and attempt to provide culturally sensitive care to both of them. He should try to meet with them separately and together to discuss their perceived family pressures. Physicians who see both partners in a relationship, however, must be very mindful of boundaries and clearly define what are shared topics versus what are individual or private issues.

References: Case 13

Bohua L. China/UNFPA Reproductive Health/Family Planning-End of Report Women Survey Report Key Finding: University of Southampton, UK, China Population Information and Research Center Division of Social Statistics, 2004 February.

Bohua L. UNFPA/CHINA Quality of Care in Reproductive Health/Family Planning Project, Fifth County Programme, Quantitative Evaluation Report, 2003–2005.

Carillo J.E., Green A.R., Betancourt J.R. Crosscultural primary care: a patient-based approach. *Ann Intern Med* 1999;130:829–34.

Higgins L.T., Zheng M., Liu Y., Sun C.H. Attitudes to marriage and sexual behaviors: a survey of gender and culture differences in China and United Kingdom: sex roles. *A J Res* 2002.

Huang W.J. An Asian perspective on relationship and marriage education. *Fam Process* 2005;44:161–73.

Key Findings. China Population & Development Research Centre, National Centre for Women and Children Health, Chinese Centre for Disease Control and Prevention and Southampton Statistical Sciences Research Institute, UK, 2006.

Kleinman A., Eisenberg L., Good B. Culture, illness and care: clinical lessons from anthropological and cross-cultural research. *Ann Intern Med* 1978; 88:251–88.

Korabik K. Women managers in the People's Republic of China: changing roles in changing times. *Appl Psychol* 1993;42:353–63.

Midlarsky E., Venkataramani-Kothari A., Plante M. Domestic violence in the Chinese and South Asian immigrant communities. *Ann N Y Acad Sci* 2006; 1087:279–300.

Morash M., Bui H., Zhang Y., Holtfreter K. Risk factors for abusive relationships: a study of Vietnamese American immigrant women. *Violence Against Women* 2007;13:653–75.

Mutha S., Allen C., Welch M. Toward culturally competent care: a toolbox for teaching communication strategies. Center for the Health Professions, University of California, San Francisco, 2002.

Raj A., Silverman J.G. Immigrant South Asian women at greater risk for injury from intimate partner violence. *Am J Public Health* 2003;93: 435–7.

Sivelle K. Chinese women and their contraceptive choices. Available at: http://www.chinadaily.com.cn/english/doc/2005-01/18/content_410003.htm.

Simmons J.A., Irwin D.B., Drinnien B.A. *Maslow's Hierarchy of Needs.* West Publishing Company, New York, 1987.

Wiebe E.R., Sent L., Fong S., Chan J. Barriers to use of oral contraceptives in ethnic Chinese women presenting for abortion. *Contraception* 2002;65: 159–63.

Wiebe E.R., Janssen P.A., Henderson A., Fung I. Ethnic Chinese women's perceptions about condoms, withdrawal and rhythm methods of birth control. *Contraception* 2004;69:493–6.

Wiebe E.R., Henderson A., Choi J., Trouton K. Ethnic Korean women's perceptions about birth control. *Contraception* 2006;73:623–7.

Wu J., Go S., Quid C. Domestic violence against women seeking induced abortion in China. *Contraception* 2005;72:117–21.

Xinxin C. Marriage Law Revisions Reflect Social Progress in China. China Today, 2001.

CASE 14

Earl Collins

A 73-year-old African American man with lung cancer

Mitchell L. Margolis, MD,[1] *and Lisa Bellini, MD*[2]

[1] Veterans Affairs Medical Center of Philadelphia, Philadelphia, PA, USA
[2] University of Pennsylvania School of Medicine, Philadelphia, PA, USA

Educational Objectives

- Explain how folk beliefs may be a very powerful component of a patient's decision making.
- Demonstrate how to engage the patient who may be using complementary or alternative medical approaches.
- Describe the important roles that religious or spiritual beliefs may play in a patient's choices regarding treatment.

TACCT Domain: 4

Case Summary, Questions and Answers

Mr. Collins is a 73-year-old African American retired mortician who is referred to Dr. Jones in a pulmonary clinic for evaluation of a lung nodule. He complains of shortness of breath with exertion but denies coughing or chest pain. He used to smoke one pack of cigarettes daily for 50 years but quit 4 months ago. His physical exam is notable for a frail elderly man with a few expiratory wheezes and moderately diminished breath sounds bilaterally. Chest x-rays over a 9-month period of a spiculated left upper lobe nodule which has grown,

---

Achieving Cultural Competency: A case-based approach to training health professionals,
1st edition. Edited by L Hark, H DeLisser. © 2009 Blackwell Publishing,
ISBN: 9781405180726.

from 1.1 × 0.9 cm to 1.9 × 1.8 cm. Tissue specimens are obtained during a subsequent bronchoscopy, which demonstrate a non-small cell lung cancer. A CT scan of the thorax and upper abdomen, MRI of the brain, and bone scan disclose no evidence of metastases, consistent with stage 1 lung cancer. He is considered to be an appropriate surgical candidate, and surgery is recommended. Mr. Collins and his wife, however, are very conflicted about surgery. In particular, they have been told by several friends that lung cancer spreads when exposed to air during surgery, and they knew a friend who had surgery for lung cancer and died a few weeks later.

1 How should lay or folk beliefs that pertain to important medical decisions be addressed?

It is essential to listen to the patients' concerns and respectfully engage them in a discussion about their beliefs. The physician has an obligation to ensure that the patient is making an informed decision and to advocate for the treatment that is felt to be in the best interest of the patient. On the other hand, a dismissive approach is much more likely to distance the physician from the patient and to make the patient less accepting of the physician's treatment recommendations.

2 How should the physician respond to this specific folk belief about air causing tumor growth or spread?

The physician can begin by acknowledging that the patient has been heard and then indicate that there are some additional things he/she would like to share. There is a widespread belief that exposing lung cancer to air at the time of surgery promotes the growth and spread of the tumor. One recent study by the American Cancer Society suggests that some of this notion may be the most prevalent misconception about cancer in the U.S. Moreover, this belief appears to be more common among African American patients compared with white patients. In developing a response to the patient who holds this belief, several things should be kept in mind.

First, belief in the hazards of exposing tumors to air may have been reinforced by personal and anecdotal experiences of the patient, which need to be identified and investigated. Second, although there is no scientific basis for the notion that exposure of a tumor to air will negatively effect the outcome, there are at least three possible mechanisms by which surgery could promote tumor growth and worsen the patient's prognosis: (i) direct seeding of the tumor to a secondary site as a result of surgical manipulation; (ii) stimulation of metastatic tumor foci by postsurgical inflammation; and (iii) accelerated metastatic tumor growth due to loss of inhibitory factors derived from the primary tumor. Furthermore, even with apparently curative surgery for stage 1 disease, about 30% of patients die within 5 years of the original operation, and tumor recurrence accounts for about 57% of these deaths.

Lastly, expression of this belief may actually reflect other unspoken concerns, such as a more general fear of surgery or distrust of the physician or medical establishment, which also needs to be explored. It is important to acknowledge these issues, while affirming the benefits of surgery. Suggested questions and responses to the patient would include:

> *"You are not alone in having this belief, as many lung cancer patients who are deciding whether or not to have lung cancer surgery have the same concern. Has this happened to someone close to you?"*

> *"In many ways what you are really asking is, 'Will the surgery itself make the cancer worse?' While there are some good scientific theories about how surgery could worsen a tumor, research tells us that you are much more likely to be alive in 5 years with surgery than without it.*

> *"What fears do you have about the surgery itself? Do you have any concerns that we might not be treating you properly?"*

Despite his misgivings, Mr. Collins eventually agrees to surgery and has a technically successful operation, although the tumor was found to comprise a 2.5 × 2.5 × 2 cm, moderate to poorly differentiated adenocarcinoma arising in a scar, with at least three smaller metastatic foci in the immediately adjacent lung parenchyma. It was decided not to administer postoperative adjuvant chemotherapy or radiotherapy because the risk-to-benefit outcome was not favorable. Several weeks later, Mr. Collins was hospitalized for hypokalemia. He admitted to Dr. Jones that he had gone to a naturopath who prescribed a "cleansing" regimen and a cocktail of "cancer-fighting" supplements, vitamins, and minerals.

3   How should Dr. Jones respond to the use of alternative medicine approaches by Mr. Collins?

CAM therapies are widely used by patients, particularly those with cancer (see Table 14.1).

The reasons why patients make use of CAM approaches are multiple and include: side effects and/or failure (perceived or real) of conventional treatments; cultural or ethnic traditions; the often distant or hurried nature of the relationships with conventional physicians; the belief that various nutritional or herbal preparations are less "processed" and thus safer and more "natural"; and suspicions of a profit motivation by the medical–hospital–pharmaceutical industry to the detriment of the health and well-being of patients.

As with folk beliefs, the physician needs to initiate a nonjudgmental respectful conversation with the patient who is employing CAM approaches. The goal is to have a relationship in which the patient is open with the physician about all aspects of his/her health. When there appears to be risk or harm, the physician is obligated to inform the patient of this fact. Guidelines on the use of nonconventional modalities that physicians can share with patients include: (i) always be knowledgeable about anything you use or take into your body; (ii) more is not always better; balance and moderation should rule; (iii) be vigilant for side effects; something is not necessarily safe because it is a "natural" product; and (iv) all of your health care

Table 14.1 Classification of CAM interventions

Alternative medical systems	Mind–body medicine	Biologic-based therapies	Manipulative and body-based methods	Energy therapies
Homeopathy Acupuncture Reflexology	Hypnosis Imagery Relaxation techniques Support groups Creative outlets (e.g. music)	Herbal dietary supplements Nonherbal dietary supplements	Massage Aromatherapy Magnet/laser therapy	Healing touch Reiki

Source: Bardia A., Barton D.L., Prokop L.J., Bauer B.A., Moynihan T.J. Efficacy of complementary and alternative medicine therapies in relieving cancer pain: a systematic review. *J Clin Oncol* 2006;24:5457–64.

providers should be aware of all of the therapeutic approaches you are using, whether they be conventional or alternative.

> *Mr. Collins was given potassium supplementation and did well for the next 12 months, but then developed neck, head, and upper extremity swelling. Thoracic MRI demonstrated extensive mediastinal adenopathy and compression of the superior vena consistent with metastatic tumor and superior vena cava syndrome. Urgent radiation therapy was indicated and strongly recommended for the patient. Mr. Collins (supported by his wife) refused this therapy, saying, "I am going to let God take care of this. If God has decided my time is up, your treatment will not really help."*

4   How should the physician respond to this religiously based refusal to accept potentially beneficial therapy?

A great premium is placed on respecting the religious beliefs and expression of patients and patients will often use their spiritual beliefs to inform their medical decisions. However, when significant medical decisions are involved, particularly when there are potentially life-threatening consequences, the physician is obligated to ensure that decisions are derived from authentic beliefs that are internally consistent and not coerced. Ultimately, this involves a respectful discussion focused on exploring these issues, which may begin with the physician but may be continued and/or completed with the patient's family, a pastoral care provider, or the patient's own spiritual advisors.

References: Case 14

Angell M., Kassirer J.P. Alternative medicine: the risks of untested and unregulated remedies. *N Engl J Med* 1998;339:839–41.

Astrow A.B., Puchalski C.M., Sulmasy D.P. Religion, spirituality, and healthcare: social ethical, and practical considerations. *Am J Med* 2001;110:283–7.

Bardia A., Barton D.L., Prokop L.J., Bauer B.A., Moynihan T.J. Efficacy of complementary and alternative medicine therapies in relieving cancer pain: a systematic review. *J Clin Oncol* 2006;24:5457–64.

Buryska J.F. Assessing the ethical eight of cultural, religious and spiritual claims in the clinical context. *J Med Ethics* 2001;27:118–22.

Dein S. Race, culture and ethnicity in minority research: a critical discussion. *J Cult Divers* 2006;13:68–75.

Detterbeck F.C., Rivera M.P., Socinski M.A., Rosenman J.G. (eds). *Diagnosis and Treatment of Lung Cancer*. WB Saunders Co. Philadelphia 2001, pp 177–90.

Gansler T., Henley S.J., Stein K., Nehl E.J., Smigal C., Slaughter E. Sociodemographic determinants of cancer treatment health literacy. *Cancer* 2005; 104:653–60.

Greene F.L., Page D.L., Fleming I.D., et al. (eds). *AJCC Cancer Staging Manual*, 6th ed. Springer, New York, 2002.

Kleinman A., Eisenberg L., Good B. Culture, illness, and care: clinical lessons from anthropological and cross-cultural research. *Ann Intern Med* 1978;88:251–88.

Margolis M.L., Christie J.D., Silvestri G.A., Kaiser L., Santiago S., Hansen-Flaschen J. Racial differences pertaining to a belief about lung cancer surgery: results of a multicenter survey. *Ann Intern Med* 2003;139:558–63.

Mountain C.F. Revisions in the international system for staging lung cancer. *Chest* 1997;111:1710–7.

Sampson W. Studying herbal remedies. *N Engl J Med* 2005;353:337–9.

Shekelle P.G., Morton S.C., Suttorp M.J., Buscemi N., Friesen C. Agency for healthcare research and quality. Challenges in systematic reviews of complementary and alternative medicine topics. *Ann Intern Med* 2005; 142:1042–7.

Strauss G.M. Clinical and pathologic factors in non-small cell lung cancer. 2007 UpToDate. Available at: http://www.uptodate.com.

Sulmasy D.P. Spiritual issues in the care of dying patients. "Its okay between me and God." *JAMA* 2006;296:1385–92.

Weiger W.A., Smith M., Boon H., Richardson M.A., Kaptchuk T.J., Eisenberg D.M. Advising patients who seek complementary and alternative medical therapies for cancer. *Ann Intern Med* 2002;137:889–903.

Wetzel M.S., Kaptchuk T.J., Haramati A., Eisenberg D.M. Complementary and alternative medical therapies: implications for medical education. *Ann Intern Med* 2003;138:191–6.

Wilson L.D., Detterbeck F., Yahalom J. Superior vena cava syndrome with malignant causes. *N Engl J Med* 2007;356:1862–9.

CASE 15

Irma Matos

A 66-year-old Ecuadorian woman with type 2 diabetes and hypertension

Edgar Maldonado, MD, and Debbie Salas-Lopez, MD, MPH, FACP
Lehigh Valley Hospital and Health Network, Allentown, PA, USA

Educational Objectives

- Learn how "dual residency" can affect a plan of care and compliance with medical treatment for diverse populations from other countries of origin.
- Describe the ease and unrestricted access to diagnostic testing and prescription drugs in Latin America, especially for travelers with U.S. currency.
- Illustrate patient patterns of travel and how this could impact the delivery of health care to a population with chronic illnesses as well as the impact of incidental and abnormal diagnostic findings from other countries, especially abnormal reports in a second language.

TACCT Domains: 1, 2, 4

Case Summary, Questions and Answers

Irma Matos is a 66-year-old Hispanic woman from Ecuador who comes to her primary care physician (PCP), Dr. Bowman, for a routine visit. Mrs. Matos immigrated to the U.S. 15 years ago to join her husband who had already been established in the U.S. for several years. She became a legal resident during this time but continues to enjoy frequent

Achieving Cultural Competency: A case-based approach to training health professionals,
1st edition. Edited by L Hark, H DeLisser. © 2009 Blackwell Publishing,
ISBN: 9781405180726.

visits to Ecuador to spend time with her two children and five grandchildren. She has a history of well-controlled type 2 diabetes and hypertension, managed with an oral hypoglycemic and an angiotensin converting enzyme (ACE) inhibitor. She also suffers from chronic lower back pain and major depression, which are treated with an anti-inflammatory (as needed) and a selective serotonin reuptake inhibitor. She worked as a housekeeper in a large hotel for 10 years, but as a result of her back pain and chronic depression, she has retired. She currently receives Medicare health care coverage.

1 How does this patient's social situation impact the care provided by Dr. Bowman?

Mrs. Matos' social situation is that she wants to spend time in Ecuador but enjoys the quality of health care provided in the U.S., which includes Medicare. Her depression may be related to the need to see her grandchildren, her chronic medical conditions, lack of acculturation, and her inability to work due to chronic back pain. Permanent resident aliens or naturalized American citizens divide their time between the United States and their country of birth. This is due in part to the ability to access a variety of health care services in the U.S. that are typically not available in their native country. In many Latin American countries, particularly Ecuador, many residents do not have health insurance and many receive health care via the public health care system, which is typically free or at low cost. However, due to the deficiencies in the public system, the services provided may not always be adequate. Consequently residents opt for private clinics or prepaid medicine that various companies in Ecuador offer with higher quality standards. In comparison to the U.S., access to doctor visits, diagnostic tests, and medications are relatively inexpensive and somewhat unregulated in Latin American countries. This allows travelers and residents to obtain diagnostic testing and medications without a doctor's prescription.

2 What additional social history is needed about Mrs. Matos' travel schedule to best manage her medical condition?

Many elderly patients from those parts of the United States that experience cold winters will spend the winter months in Southern states such as Florida. Similarly, patients originally from warm weather climates, such as South America, the Caribbean, and

Table 15.1 Questions to ask patients about traveling

- What is nature of your traveling? (Depending on your relationship with the patient, he/she might or might not let you know.)
- What is your planned duration or length of stay?
- Who will you be staying with?
- Do you have a primary care doctor there in case of an emergency?
- What kind of activities will you be involved in? (especially if touring or walking long distances. This is very important for patients who may not recognize their physical limitations, are at risk for falls, or are on insulin that may need adjusting.)
- Are you preparing the meals? Will you have access to a supermarket?
- What kinds of problems or barriers might be encountered that would lead to interruption of your usual care plan?
- Is there a knowledgeable caregiver or contact who may assist with medications, management of medical conditions, and continuation of care plan during your visit?
- Do you have a plan in place to obtain medication refills?
- Have you obtained travel information on outbreaks and endemic diseases, and did you receive the necessary vaccinations or prophylaxis as recommended by the CDC (http://www.cdc/gov/travel)?

Source: Edgar Maldonado, MD, Lehigh Valley Hospital, 2009. Used with permission

Mexico, will frequently spend the entire winter season living in their native country. By anticipating and considering this pattern, the physician can incorporate their travel plans into their plan of care. This will also help identify, in a proactive manner, potential problems that patients may encounter and will improve continuity of care. These include running out of medications, inability to adhere to prescribed or recommended diets, or decline in self-management skills. Questions to ask patients about traveling are shown in Table 15.1.

Three months later, Mrs. Matos returns to her PCP, Dr. Bowman. She explains that she returned from Ecuador last week but ran out of her diabetes and hypertension medications during the last 2 weeks of her trip. At this visit, she presents with polydypsia, polyuria, blurred vision, and fatigue, and her prescriptions are renewed. Her blood pressure is also noted to be elevated and, on review of systems, she is positive for multiple vegetative signs of depression. She was scheduled to see her mental health care provider last month but missed her appointment because she was out of the country. She is encouraged to reschedule this appointment. Mrs. Matos also informs Dr. Bowman that she "felt ill" at the beginning of her vacation and visited the local "policlinic." For unknown reasons, the physician requested that she have a repeat colonoscopy, ultrasound of kidneys and gallbladder, ECG, and some blood tests. She tells Dr. Bowman that she thought she needed a CT scan of the brain because she was having headaches. Mrs. Matos shows Dr. Bowman these reports, which are in Spanish, and asks her to review and interpret the results because "no one had explained the results to her."

3 What might be done to prevent Mrs. Matos from running out of her medications during future trips to Ecuador?

Medicare/Medicaid generally provide for a 1-month supply of medications at one time, unless the patient is on vacation. Only then will they provide up to a 60-day supply, but only one time per year. Therefore, as part of travel planning, the physician needs to make sure that the patient has a process in place in the U.S. to obtain his/her medication refills in a timely manner. The best approach that seems to work for many patients is having a friend or relative obtain the refills and medical supplies (test strips, lancets, etc.) and mail them promptly to the patient. Keep in mind that, with many prescription plans, patients can only get refills 7 days before they are due, and it may take up to 10 or more days for medications to reach their destination in foreign countries. Timing is therefore extremely important when medications are life-sustaining and require special handling, such as insulin which requires refrigeration. Another way is to use mail-order scripts that provide a 90-day supply of medications. During travel, airport security restrictions apply and medications should only be stored in a carry-on bag in labeled bottles to avoid treatment interruption, if and when, checked luggage is lost or delayed.

4 What are some of the reasons for why these tests may have been ordered?

Many patients who return from Latin American countries with test results tell their physicians that they initiated the request because they were concerned about their health, or were advised by a family member to get further evaluation. In addition, this may also be a manifestation of a dissatisfaction or skepticism over the recommendations or care provided by the U.S. physician. The self-initiation of testing or treatment also in part reflects the culture and how health care is organized in some parts of Latin America. In Ecuador, for those who can afford it, there is the cultural expectation that comprehensive evaluations will always be undertaken, even for common ailments. In addition, studies such as CT scans and ultrasounds can be done there without a physician referral and paid for with U.S. currency. Further, in some Latin American countries, medical care, diagnostic tests, and surgical procedures are less expensive than in the U.S. and are readily accessible for travelers. This may cause visiting patients to perceive that healthcare is more affordable and easier to access in some of these countries. Added to all of this is the fact that in some parts of Ecuador many physicians generate income from the variety of tests offered at their medical centers or "policlinics". These entities sometimes compete and market to the consumer, promoting early detection of various diseases which some patients may not be at risk for. Websites for diagnostic centers may state "No one is exempt from becoming ill. Early disease detection is the best way to save your life". Clinics offer packages, such as "Paquete de examenes de prevencion general" translated as "general prevention packet", which includes a battery of blood tests, x-rays, ultrasound, EKG, pap smear, urine and stool analysis for a fraction of the cost in the U.S. This was certainly the case for Mrs. Matos on this visit to Ecuador. Given all this, it is not surprising that when patients such as Mrs. Matos return to the United States, they will have with them the results of several diagnostic tests that may not have been indicated.

With respect to Mrs. Matos, when she complained of headaches, her daughter advised her to get a CT scan of the brain "to make sure she did not have a brain tumor." And although she had had a normal screening colonoscopy a year ago, she had a repeat study in Ecuador since it was offered for a very affordable price.

5 What might Dr. Bowman do to minimize the likelihood that Mrs. Matos will seek unnecessary diagnostic studies while abroad?

Having had these experiences with Mrs. Matos, it would be important for Dr. Bowman at a visit to question Mrs. Matos about any upcoming, extended visits to Ecuador. If a trip is planned then the following should be done:
• Confirm that the patient is in a stable condition for travel;
• Review and refill medications;

- Provide the patient with a medical history summary, medication list, and allergies in case of a medical emergency;
- Ensure that the patient is up to date on vaccinations and has other prophylaxis medications prior to travel; or
- Develop strategies for the patient to communicate with the office or physician when they are out of the country (phone, email, family).

This is an ideal time to identify and anticipate any potential problems, to emphasize the importance of adherence to their medical plan, and to answer questions in regard to management of potential complications during travel.

6   How do changes in the diet and lifestyle of Mrs. Matos while in Ecuador affect her diabetes and hypertension management?

Patients who spend a significant amount of time in their native country often revert back to their preexisting diet and lifestyle patterns. This may or may not be an advantage, depending on where they live, what they do, and who is preparing the meals. Patients sometimes get caught up with festivities and family gatherings, especially during holidays. This could lead to excess caloric, carbohydrate, or salt intake and alcohol consumption. Some will also stop medications if they are planning to consume alcohol, which could result in acute complications. An interesting paradox is that some patients might actually lose weight as they feel more comfortable and at ease walking in warmer climates and to known local destinations (internal tourism), in contrast to an often more sedentary lifestyle in the U.S.

The Ecuadorian diet or cuisine varies from region to region, but like many Latin American countries, Ecuador's daily diet is based on rice, soups, corn, and bananas. Meals on the coast will have a great variety of seafood which, if poorly prepared in their signature dish "ceviche," could be a source of food-borne illness. Natural juices made from exotic fruits like passion fruit, tree tomato, guanabana, blackberry, and papaya are very popular. This often results in elevated blood sugar in diabetics. When on vacation, many look forward to these foods, particularly the fruit drinks. It is very challenging to change their diet especially when on vacation, as many of them do not have control over how meals are prepared. They do have control over portion size, which in the absence of calorie counting is a good way to maintain a balanced diet, yet still sample the food.

> One month later, Mrs. Matos returns to the clinic and tells Dr. Bowman that she has been taking her medications but that her blood sugar still seems to be high when she tests it in the morning. She explains to Dr. Bowman that her sister, who has osteoarthritis, gave her a medication that makes her back feel better. She shows Dr. Bowman the pill and asks her to prescribe this medication today and says she finds it convenient when her family, friends, and local pharmacist give her medications without a doctor's prescription. Dr. Bowman identifies this medication as a steroid/anti-inflammatory combination medication, which partially explains why her diabetes is uncontrolled despite taking her oral hypoglycemic medication.

7   How should Dr. Bowman approach Mrs. Matos' request to prescribe a steroid combination pill for her back pain which she self-prescribed in Ecuador?

It is not uncommon for patients traveling to Latin America to have unrestricted access to prescription drugs. Many countries have their own pharmaceutical companies that make medications and combinations not found or dispensed in the U.S. The relatively high proportion of drugs dispensed without a medical prescription that nevertheless require medical follow-up, such as diabetes medications, probably reflects limited access to medical care. In many cases, these combination drugs are generics used to treat chronic conditions like diabetes, arthritis, and high blood pressure. These medications are inexpensive and can be obtained at street markets or pharmacies without a prescription.

Unlike the U.S., in Ecuador and many other Latin American countries, it is legally permissable for pharmacists to diagnose and give medical treatment without a physician's prescription. Sharing medications among family members is a common practice in the U.S. as well as in many Latin America countries and is usually done by an adult maternal figure or community member that the family trusts for medical advice. Many times this person has several chronic conditions him/herself and therefore has access to medications and household remedies and has more experience with health care than other members of the household or community.

Table 15.2 Travel chart summary items

- Patient demographics
- Emergency contact in the U.S. and the visiting country
- Allergies
- Active medical problems
- Inactive medical problems
- Medications
- Immunization record
- Pharmacy information
- Primary care physician contact information, including after-hours number

---

Source: Edgar Maldonado, MD, Lehigh Valley Hospital, 2009. Used with permission.

8   How can the medical care of patients living in the U.S. and abroad, such as Mrs. Matos, be improved?

First and foremost, patient education and self-management training should include travel planning and cover self-prescribing practices. Physicians need information and understanding about their patients' culture and health beliefs and the health care system in their native country. A reasonable way to improve the medical care for "dual-residents" is to incorporate their travel plans and travel health into their plan of care. A multidisciplinary approach (case managers, patient navigators, or nursing staff) with input from the physician is an effective strategy to use. Patients would benefit from an understanding that, although they might see it as an extended vacation, they still need to adhere to their nutrition regimen as well as medical treatment. A process for obtaining medication refills should be in place if traveling for more than 30 days. Patients should travel with a summary of medical conditions, allergies, vaccinations, and an updated medication list with dosing information (as shown in Table 15.2).

References: Case 15

Besson M. Self-medication amongst illegal Latino-American Immigrants: necessary or inappropriate. *Rev Med Suisse* 2007;3(127):2239–43.

Centers for Disease Control and Prevention. Travelers' health. Available at: http://www.cdc.gov/travel/.

Drug Utilization Research Group, Latin America. Multicenter study on self-medication and self-prescription in six Latin American countries. *Clin Pharmacol Therapeut* 1997;61(4):488–93.

Fleitas I. The quality of radiology services in five Latin American countries. *Rev Panam Salud Publica* 2006;20(2-3):113–24.

Understanding Supplemental Security Income Continuing Disability Reviews. Social Security Administration Online, 2007 Edition. Available at: http://www.ssa.gov.

World Health Organization. Guidelines for the regulatory assessment of medicinal products for use in self-medication. World Health Organization, Geneva, 2000:9.

CASE 16

Eileen Clark

An 82-year-old African American woman with a stroke

Scott Kasner, MD, and Horace DeLisser, MD
University of Pennsylvania School of Medicine, Philadelphia, PA, USA

Educational Objectives

- Describe cultural factors that may impact the process of informed consent.
- Identify factors that enhance the likelihood of a good outcome when there is suspicion and distrust.
- Examine the impact of the Tuskegee Syphilis Study on the practice of medicine and biomedical research.
- Review the importance of honest, open, and ongoing communication.

TACCT Domains: 1, 3, 4

Case Summary, Questions and Answers

Mrs. Clark is an 82-year-old African American woman with hypertension who collapses at home with right-sided weakness and inability to speak. Her family initially put her in bed and tried to get her to take her blood pressure medications, but she was unable to swallow. When she did not improve after several hours, emergency medical services was called and she was transported to the Emergency Department (ED). In the ED, an acute stroke is strongly suspected, although the initial CT scan was

---

Achieving Cultural Competency: A case-based approach to training health professionals,
1st edition. Edited by L Hark, H DeLisser. © 2009 Blackwell Publishing,
ISBN: 9781405180726.

> normal. The stroke team is called and agrees with the diagnosis of a probable acute stroke, but determines that too much time (>8 hours) has elapsed for her to receive thrombolytic therapy. Dr. Stuart Kottler, the head of the stroke team, is currently an investigator in a clinical trial to assess the efficacy of a potential new stroke medication. He approaches the patient's 55-year-old son and four grandchildren, saying, "It is too late for standard therapy, but she may be eligible to participate in a research study using a new medication. Unlike standard therapy, this medication can be used for up to 12 hours after a stroke. Timing is critical, though, so we do not have much more time to make a decision."
>
> The son responds, "Why do you want to treat my mother like a guinea pig? What are you really going to do to help her?"

1 What would be an appropriate response to this question?

Most Americans, regardless of their race or ethnicity, are typically hesitant about participating in a research study or using an experimental medication because of a concern that things might not be done in their best interest or for their well-being. These fears may be more pronounced in Blacks, because of the well-documented abuse that occurred in the Tuskegee Syphilis Study, which has had a tremendous impact on the collective psyche of a large number of African Americans. It has led to an undercurrent of suspicion toward medicine in general, and biomedical research in particular, and has been one of the factors that has hampered the recruitment of African Americans into clinical trials, particularly those involving HIV and AIDS. The underrepresentation of blacks in these studies, in turn, may contribute to health-related disparities, since the results may not be generalizable to understudied populations who do not have access to novel therapies. These cultural dynamics need to be kept in mind as physicians seek consent, not just for a clinical trial, but for any medical intervention. Given the various governmental responses to address the abuses of the Tuskegee study, some clinicians may believe that this study should be viewed as a sad historical occurrence that is no longer relevant. However, the data pointing to undertreatment and the evidence of institutional racism mean fear of exploitation and abuse will continue to be issues of concern for a significant number of patients from minority communities.

With these issues in mind, the goal is to obtain informed consent in a way that accurately represents the trial without using coercive or manipulative language. Respect, patience, truthfulness, and a genuine effort to listen and respond to patients' concerns will go a long way to ensuring a good outcome when issues of race may be part of the dynamic. Further, it is important to avoid responding with anger or defensiveness if the motivations of the physicians or institution are questioned. It is also helpful to stress that the patient will receive the best possible care regardless of the decision that is made. It is useful to recognize that patients and their families appreciate hearing, in plain language, the benefits rather than a focus on the risk of the treatment or procedure. Lastly, although the goal is to recruit the patient into the research study, if the patient or family declines to participate, they should know that all potential treatment options have been fully considered.

Tuskegee Syphilis Study

The Tuskegee study, a Public Health-sponsored observational study of the effects of untreated syphilis on African American men, is now recognized as one of the saddest and most regrettable enterprises in biomedical research. The study was launched in 1932 at the Tuskegee Institute in Alabama, using African American men with untreated latent syphilis to document the presence or absence of destructive syphilitic lesions. In 1932, standard treatment consisted only of potentially toxic arsenic agents, whose effectiveness was questionable. At the time, it was widely believed that there were racial differences in the natural history of syphilis, supposedly more benign in blacks. This study aimed, in part, to generate data that would challenge that belief and thus support efforts to increase governmental funding of public health efforts targeted at blacks. The study consisted of 399 poor black men with syphilis, along with 201 controls, and was originally designed to last only 6 to 9 months.

The study, however, took on a life of its own and continued until it was terminated in 1973 following its disclosure in the press. By that time, 28 of the men had died directly from syphilis; 100 were dead from associated complications; 40 of their wives had become infected; and 19 of their children had been born with congenital syphilis. Even judged by the standards of the time, the study was problematic on a number of fronts. By labeling their diagnosis as "bad blood," a term used by black people in the rural south to describe a variety of ailments, study participants were led to believe they had something other than a venereal disease. Potentially coercive incentives such as free physical examinations, food, and transportation were used to induce participation in the study.

Lumbar punctures were misrepresented as treatment and were performed without local anesthesia. And although effective antibiotics for the treatment of latent syphilis became available in the 1940s, the syphilitic subjects were not informed of this treatment, and extreme measures were often taken to ensure that they did not receive antibiotic therapy.

The continuance of this study over 40 years was driven by investigators who saw a unique scientific "opportunity" to acquire data, and was enabled by well-meaning, but naïve black health care providers and community institutions. The study also would not have been possible if not for the poverty of Macon county; the lack of adequate health care in the area; and the trusting nature of the community that made these men vulnerable to deception, exploitation, and manipulation. Certainly this kind of research endeavor could only have continued for four decades in the context of societal and institutional racisms that did not acknowledge the humanity of these men.

The knowledge of this study and its abuses has had a profound impact on much of the collective psyche of African Americans and has helped to reinforce distrust and suspicion of physicians and medicine in general. These feelings have been further increased by the widespread misbelief that the Tuskegee men were part of an experiment in which they were injected with syphilis. Discontent and anger around the Tuskegee study has helped to fuel beliefs in the African American community that AIDS is a man-made disease intentionally inflected on blacks for the purpose of genocide. This, in turn, has led to resistance to HIV education programs and other efforts to limit the spread of HIV among African Americans. Knowledge of this study and a resulting fear of abuse have also contributed to unwillingness on the part of many African Americans to participate in clinical trials.

One of Mrs. Clark's granddaughters then asks, "How do you know if this new drug will work in an elderly African American woman?"

---

2   What would be an appropriate response to this question?

For these kinds of situations, where there is suspicion or distrust, the most effective approach is one of honesty, openness, and truthfulness. A possible response might be:

> *"That is an excellent question. To be honest, this drug has only been studied in a relatively small number of people. In these studies, the drug does appear to be safe and potentially effective, but there were very*

few African American patients enrolled in the studies. This is precisely why we have approached you. Stroke affects people of all ages and races, particularly African Americans, and so we feel it is important that we include patients, such as your mother and grandmother, in these studies. This is the only way to find out if this medication works in general, regardless of things like age, race, or gender."

As the discussion continues it becomes clear that, although her son is comfortable giving consent, the grandchildren are uncomfortable with her participation in the study.

3   As time is critical, how do you get consensus among family members?

The conversation must begin with a clear and concise description of the patient's condition and the relevant treatment options that enables real understanding on the part of the family. First, ask the family how they make medical decisions, and second, what is their understanding of what is going on and what options exist. Active listening instead of telling or speaking is more time effective because it affords the clinician the opportunity to query health literacy levels, expectations, and understanding. It is often helpful to reframe the information several times, and then use that understanding to frame the conversation in terms of how the patient had lived her life and the values and beliefs she had. This is particularly important because families in times of medical crises may tend to make decisions in terms of their fears, guilt, grief, anger, etc. Negotiating and affirming the difficulty of handling emotions is as important as the content of the message. So, at this point, Dr. Kottler may have said:

"I need you to first think about who your mother and grandmother was before she had this stroke. And then imagine if she could, in fact, speak for herself. What would she want for herself? What do you think she would say?"

After nearly 45 minutes of discussion with the physicians and among themselves, the family agreed that it would be in the best interest of Mrs. Clark to participate in the trial.

4 Now that you have consent, how do you maintain this rapport with the family?

Having developed rapport and gained some measure of trust (at least enough to obtain consent), it is important to continue to actively build on this relationship between the health care team and the family. Trust is maintained and supported when the communication from the physician to the patient and/or family is goal-oriented and patient-centered, understandable, jargon-free, truthful, honest, timely, and consistent. Communicating effectively in this way will go a long way toward building the kind of trust that helps to prevent conflicts or misunderstandings over care.

References: Case 16

Corbie-Smith G. The continuing legacy of the Tuskegee Syphilis Study: considerations for clinical investigation. *Am J Med Sci* 1999;317:5–8.

Corbie-Smith G., Thomas S.B., Williams M.V., Moody-Ayers S. Attitudes and beliefs of African-Americans toward participation in medical research. *J Gen Intern Med* 1999;14:537–46.

Fairchild A.L., Bayer R. Uses and abuses of Tuskegee. *Science* 1999;284(5416): 919–21.

Gray J.D. The problem of consent in emergency medicine research. *Can J Emerg Med* 2001;3:213–8.

Green D., Rickles F.R. Enhancing participation in clinical research: keys to obtaining informed consent. *J Support Oncol* 2007;5:48–50.

Guinan M.E. Black communities' belief in "AIDS as genocide". A barrier to overcome for HIV prevention. *Ann Epidemiol* 1993;3:193–5.

Jones J. *Bad Blood: The Tuskegee Syphilis Experiment–A tragedy of Race and Medicine.* The Free Press, New York, 1993.

Levine C., Zuckerman C. The trouble with families: toward an ethic of accommodation. *Ann Intern Med* 1999;130:148–52.

Levinson W., Roter D.L., Mullooly J.P., Dull V.T., Frankel R.M. Physician-patient communication: the relationship with malpractice claims among primary care physicians and surgeons. *JAMA* 1997;277:553–9.

Shavers V.L., Lynch C.F., Burmeister L.F. Factors that influence African-Americans' willingness to participate in medical research studies. *Cancer* 2001;91(1):233–6 (suppl).

Shavers V.L., Lynch C.F., Burmeister L.F. Racial differences in factors that influence the willingness to participate in medical research studies. *Ann Epidemiol* 2002;12:248–56.

Sheikh A. Why are ethnic minorities underrepresented in U.S. research studies? *PLoS Med* 2006;3(2):e19.

Smith-Tytler J. Informed consent, confidentiality, and subject rights in clinical trials. *Proc Am Thorac Soc* 2007;4:189–93.

Stephenson A.C., Baker S., Zeps N. Attitudes of relatives of patients in intensive care and emergency departments to surrogate consent to research on incapacitated participants. *Crit Care Resusc* 2007;9:40–50.

Stewart M., Brown J.B., Boon H., Galajda J., Meredith L., Sangster M. Evidence on patient-doctor communication. *Cancer Prev Control* 1999;3:25–30.

Thomas S.B., Quinn S.C. The Tuskegee Syphilis Study, 1932 to 1972: implications for HIV education and AIDS risk education programs in the black community. *Am J Public Health* 1991;81:1498–505.

Wendler D., Kington R., Madans J., et al. Are racial and ethnic minorities less willing to participate in health research? *PLoS Med* 2006;3(2):e19.

White R.M. Unraveling the Tuskegee study of untreated syphilis. *Arch Intern Med* 2000;160:585–98.

White-Bateman S.R., Schumacher H.C., Sacco R.L., Appelbaum P.S. Consent for intravenous thrombolysis in acute stroke: review and future directions. *Arch Neurol* 2007;64:785–92.

CASE 17

Leslie O'Malley

A 66-year-old Irish American man with breast cancer

J. Eric Russell, MD

University of Pennsylvania School of Medicine, Philadelphia, PA, USA

Educational Objectives

- Describe how stereotyping can negatively impact the patient–physician relationship.
- Demonstrate how a patient's gender can influence his/her response to illness.
- Analyze how ethnicity can affect family dynamics that are involved in end-of-life decision-making processes.

TACCT Domains: 3, 4, 6

Case Summary, Questions and Answers

Mr. Leslie O'Malley is a 66-year-old Irish-born U.S. citizen who presents as a new patient to Dr. Beck, a primary care physician (PCP), after feeling a lump in his right breast. He denies nipple discharge, axillary masses, weight loss, fever, or chills. His past medical history is notable only for mild hypertension. Mr. O'Malley has not smoked in more than 20 years and reports social alcohol use. A focused examination demonstrates bilateral gynecomastia and confirms the presence of a right breast mass. Laboratory studies are obtained in the office. Mr. O'Malley is provided a referral for a mammogram and scheduled for a follow-up appointment

Achieving Cultural Competency: A case-based approach to training health professionals,
1st edition. Edited by L Hark, H DeLisser. © 2009 Blackwell Publishing,
ISBN: 9781405180726.

in 1 week. Mr. O'Malley returns for his follow-up appointment as planned but has failed to schedule a mammogram as instructed. His laboratory studies are entirely normal with the exception of an isolated mild elevation in his plasma bilirubin level. Dr. Beck interprets the combination of gynecomastia and elevated bilirubin as indicating potentially heavy alcohol consumption and asks the patient, "How much alcohol do you really drink?" Mr. O'Malley denies significant use of alcohol, insisting that he drinks no more than two beers a week. Dr. Beck, however, continues to press the issue, asking, "Are you sure? Are you absolutely sure? It's okay to admit the truth." Mr. O'Malley responds angrily, "Why do you keep asking me? I already told you the truth: I only drink socially."

1 Why might Dr. Beck have doubted Mr. O'Malley's self-reported alcohol consumption?

The Irish are commonly portrayed as a hard-drinking, hard-living people. Demographic studies suggest that Irish immigrants are no more likely to consume alcohol than indigenous groups, although those who do drink may do so in higher amounts. Whereas alcohol use can be associated with gynecomastia and liver function abnormalities, an isolated elevation in plasma bilirubin would be unusual. Although Dr. Beck may have some clinical basis for suspecting that Mr. O'Malley is underreporting his alcohol use, ethnic stereotypes may have led him to challenge the patient's drinking history more aggressively. Although "stereotyping" may be an unconscious reflex reaction by a physician during the diagnostic process, it carries significant risks, including the introduction of mistrust into the doctor–patient relationship. The difference between a hypothesis and a stereotype is that a hypothesis asks questions to see if they are germane, while stereotyping looks for attributes that support preformed opinions. Stereotypes are ill-filtering descriptions put on people by others and are impervious to experience or data. Without experience or exposures, general guidelines or behavior within groups are commonly considered first. This situation might have been avoided if Dr. Beck had first stated his reasons for pursuing Mr. O'Malley's drinking history, then rephrased his questions in a nonjudgmental way.

Mr. O'Malley reluctantly schedules a mammogram for the following week. His wife accompanies him to the clinic, where Mr. O'Malley registers at the front desk and is instructed to take a seat with other

*patients in a small adjoining waiting room. After a short wait, a technol-
ogist enters the waiting area and asks, "Is Leslie O'Malley here?" When
Mr. O'Malley stands, the technologist states, "Not you, sir, just your
wife." Embarrassed, Mr. O'Malley responds, "I am Leslie O'Malley, and
I am here for a mammogram." The scene is witnessed by many other
women in the small waiting area. Mr. O'Malley is escorted to a dressing area where he puts on a hospital gown, then he is escorted to a
smaller area to await his examination. Mr. O'Malley is the only male in
this room. Several minutes later, he is greeted by a technician who introduces herself and comments, "Wow, you're my first guy." Later, in the
mammogram suite, she jokingly remarks, "Looks like an A cup; hope I
can do this right." The following day Dr. Beck calls Mr. O'Malley to inform him that a suspicious mass has been detected in the right breast.
Dr. Beck outlines a diagnostic plan beginning with a needle biopsy of
the mass. Mr. O'Malley abruptly hangs up on Dr. Beck, refuses to answer several follow-up calls over the next 3 days, and fails to make the
recommended arrangements for a diagnostic needle biopsy.*

2   Why might Mr. O'Malley have refused the recommended diagnostic procedure?

Patients facing a possible diagnosis of cancer may sometimes be
reluctant to obtain critical diagnostic procedures. Mr. O'Malley's
decision may have been further complicated by his public embarrassment while awaiting his mammogram. Gender may influence
the meaning and significance of several diagnoses, including breast
cancer, which is relatively uncommon in men. Whereas a woman's
response to a breast cancer diagnosis might include fear of disfiguring
surgery, a man's response might center on issues of gender-identity
and a perceived loss of masculinity. Men may also exhibit difficulty
in coping with the loss of independence, particularly in the setting
of chronic and/or terminal conditions.

Breast Cancer in Men

Breast cancer is an uncommon disease in men. The age frequency dis-
tribution in women with breast cancer is bimodal with peaks at 52 and
71 years, whereas in men, it is unimodal with a peak at age 71 years.
Clinically, male breast cancer is similar to postmenopausal breast cancer in women. Delay in diagnosis often results from ignorance of the

existence of breast cancer among men. This, in turn, negatively affects prognosis, which has improved very little over the past three decades. The management of male breast cancer has been largely derived from randomized trials performed in women.

Eight months later, Mr. O'Malley agrees to a needle biopsy, which confirms that his breast mass (which has enlarged significantly) is malignant. Subsequent evaluation demonstrates the presence of numerous large metastatic lesions in his lungs and bone. Following a unilateral mastectomy, Mr. O'Malley receives first-line chemotherapy but fails to achieve a significantly clinical response. Following his last scheduled cycle of chemotherapy, Mr. O'Malley is admitted for chemotherapy-induced neutropenia and pneumonia that progresses to respiratory failure requiring intubation and mechanical ventilation. His condition deteriorates, and on hospital day 10, Mr. O'Malley develops acute renal failure. At the same time, he develops cognitive dysfunction, requiring the medical staff to discuss the risks and benefits of dialysis treatment with Mr. O'Malley's family. The family is advised that, even with dialysis, the probability that Mr. O'Malley will recover to the point that he could leave the hospital is less than 10%. Mrs. O'Malley and her oldest son argue that Mr. O'Malley has suffered enough and that it is time to "let him go." The patient's three daughters and youngest son, however, strongly believe that their father needs to be given every chance to recover and, as Catholics, they believe that they are required to make every effort to preserve their father's life.

---

3 What role should the physician play in mediating this end-of-life dispute? How should issues of religion and spirituality be included in the decision-making process?

The ethnicity of a family can impact how conflicts are resolved and how decisions are made. It is essential that physicians consider this factor when participating in surrogate decision-making processes. Nursing, pastoral care, and social work staff may be particularly helpful in gauging this aspect of the family dynamic and in reminding the family that decisions should be based on what the patient (not the family) would likely desire, based on his/her stated wishes, relevant experiences, and personal values. It is also important to recognize that a patient's personal values may differ significantly from the values corresponding to his/her stated religion. For example, invoking Catholic theology is relevant only if this tradition was still meaningful to Mr. O'Malley. Moreover, it is not uncommon for an individual to be confused or ignorant about the beliefs of his/her religious faith, leading to misstatements or misrepresentation of those beliefs. To confirm the accuracy of religious assertions, it may be helpful to involve pastoral care staff or to suggest that the family discuss relevant issues with clergy from their faith.

Catholicism and End-of-Life Issues

In the Catholic faith, the relationship between a patient and a physician is considered a "covenant" built on the intrinsic good of humankind. This goodness is defined by a universal morality that is often referred to as "natural law." The Church explains that the fifth commandment, "Thou shalt not kill," is a direct corollary of natural law and thus defines man's moral obligation to perform whatever act feasible to preserve life. In the case of end-of-life medical decision making, the lines between life and death, treatment and suffering, are often blurred. In this case, it is the duty of the physician to provide his/her patient with all treatment options and to assess each option with a risk:benefit ratio. The patient and his family have the right to distinguish between "ordinary" and "extraordinary" treatment options in order to make their decision.

The Catholic Church defines "ordinary" options as those that preserve health without causing undue harm to the patient. Examples include providing the patient with food, fluids, and standard medical care. "Extraordinary" options are those that will cause the patient excessive pain, sorrow, financial burden, or offer little benefit to the patient's long-term health outcome. The ultimate decision as to whether a treatment option is "ordinary" or "extraordinary" is left to the patient and his family's discretion. It is often advised that a patient and his family seek the assistance of a priest or other moral theologian when making decisions bearing on this matter. Generally speaking, providing a patient with food and water is considered an "ordinary" and morally necessary act. However, the Church defines times when this act is no longer obligatory. Providing normal care, however, is always a moral obligation. Because suicide is an immoral act under this faith system, the Church is careful to explain that refusal of additional treatment, if the results would offer no additional benefit, is *not* a form of suicide. Therefore, if a patient's condition has deteriorated to the point where nourishment no longer provides benefit, withholding food for the comfort of the patient becomes a morally correct action.

References: Case 17

Buryska J.F. Assessing the ethical eight of cultural, religious and spiritual claims in the clinical context. *J Med Ethics* 2001;27:118–122.

Donovan T., Flynn M. What makes a man a man? The lived experience of male breast cancer. *Cancer Nurs* 2007;30:464–70.

Fentiman I.S., Fourquet A., Hortobagyi G.N. Male breast cancer. *Lancet* 2006;367:595–604.

Giordano S.H., Cohen D.S., Buzdar A.U., Perkins G., Hortobagyi G.N. Breast carcinoma in men: a population-based study. *Cancer* 2004;101:51–7.

Greenslade L., Pearson M., Madden M. A good man's fault: alcohol and Irish people at home and abroad. *Alcohol* 1995;30:407–17.

Harasymiw J., Seaberg J., Bean P. Using routine laboratory tests to detect heavy drinking in the general population. *J Addict Dis* 2006;25(2):59–63.

Montalto N.J., Bean P. Use of contemporary biomarkers in the detection of chronic alcohol use. *Med Sci Monit* 2003;9:RA285–90.

Mullen K., Williams R., Hunt K. Irish descent, religion, and alcohol and tobacco use. *Addiction* 1996;91:243–54.

National Catholic Bioethics Center. A Catholic Guide to End-of-Life Decisions. Available at: http://www.ncbcenter.org/eol.asp.

Ravandi-Kashani F., Hayes T.G. Male breast cancer: a review of the literature. *Eur J Cancer* 1998;34:1341–7.

Sillanaukee P. Laboratory markers of alcohol abuse. *Alcohol* 1996;31:613–6.

Sulmasy D.P. Spiritual issues in the care of dying patients. "Its okay between me and God". *JAMA* 2006;296:1385–92.

Vig E.K., Taylor J.S., Starks H., Hopley E.K., Fryer-Edwards K. Beyond substituted judgment: how surrogates navigate end-of-life decision-making. *J Am Geriatr Soc* 2006;54:1688–93.

CASE 18

Juana Caban

A 21-year-old Puerto Rican woman who is pregnant and HIV-positive

Lisa Rucker, MD, Nadine T. Katz, MD, and Nicholas E.S. Sibinga, MD
Albert Einstein College of Medicine, Bronx, NY, USA

Educational Objectives

- Identify the cultural influences that may affect patients' requests.
- Define and express ethical precepts of veracity, autonomy, and beneficence and how they impact care in some situations.
- Identify and analyze the social stressors and the described effects of acculturation on family dynamics and beliefs.
- Discuss the ethical and legal implications of providing false information or withholding information in a clinical situation.

TACCT Domains: 2, 3, 4, 6

Case Summary, Questions and Answers

Juana Caban is a 21-year-old Puerto Rican American female who lives with her mother, Isabella Caban. Juana discovers that she is pregnant using a home pregnancy test and makes an appointment at the obstetrical clinic at the local hospital several weeks later. She is seen by Dr. Paul Graham, a first-year resident in obstetrics and gynecology. Juana is found to be 5 months

Achieving Cultural Competency: A case-based approach to training health professionals,
1st edition. Edited by L Hark, H DeLisser. © 2009 Blackwell Publishing,
ISBN: 9781405180726.

> pregnant and has not received previous prenatal care. This is her first
> pregnancy. She has been previously healthy, takes no prescribed medica-
> tions, and denies smoking, alcohol, or drug use. Juana attended public
> high school, graduating three years ago. She works as a cashier and part-
> time stocker in a small neighborhood grocery store while she considers
> whether or not to attend college. Dr. Graham, whose parents are both
> physicians and who is now the father of an infant son himself, discusses
> the difficulties in finding the best private day care setting for her baby
> and asks her what the father of the baby does for a living.

1 What might we erroneously assume about Juana's social and economic network?

What an individual comes to see and accept as "traditional" and normative is a product of his/her personal social context. Dr. Graham appears to be from a stable home with two parents and an upper middle class background. This frame of reference may have led to inaccurate assumptions that the baby's father is involved and that Juana has disposable income for day care. Assuming that the father is still a part of the patient's life and that he will be present at the birth, help raise the child, and provide financial and emotional support may lead to errors of omission in obtaining the patient's history.

Instead, it would have been much more helpful for Dr. Graham to have asked a series of questions (shown in Table 18.1) that would aid in clarifying the patient's attitude toward the pregnancy, her social support and need for additional assistance, as well as screen for possible abuse or the need for sexual safety planning.

In fact, the father of Juana's baby is no longer involved with Juana and has not participated in any of the pregnancy decision making, nor will he be providing any financial support.

2 Describe how you would obtain information about Juana's support system for her pregnancy, birth, and care of the baby?

A high percentage of all births in urban settings are to single, teenage mothers, and as a result, the mother of the patient (eventual grandmother) may play a more active role in raising the child. Many single, pregnant women are in their teens and the daughter of a teenage mother is at greater risk of becoming a pregnant teenager.

Table 18.1 Questions for physicians to ask pregnant women

- How do you feel about this pregnancy?
- Who have you told about the pregnancy?
- Is the baby's father still part of your life? (*If not, consider whether she was raped and always consider sexually transmitted diseases.*)
- Is the baby's father aware that you are pregnant?
- Do you think he will be involved with the baby?

Source: Ana Núñez, MD, Drexel University School of Medicine, and Darwin Deen, MD, Sophie Davis College of Biomedical Science, 2009. Used with permission.

Because Juana will need support through her pregnancy, the physician needs to find out about her mother and other family support. There are many kinds of families beyond the nuclear, heterosexual, two-parent home. Physicians need to explore these areas by asking, "Who lives at home with you? Is your family able to help you with this pregnancy? If yes, who all do you mean (asking for names and family roles) could be involved?"

In this case, because Juana lives with her mother, it would be helpful to ask her questions directly to get an understanding of her relationship with her mother. Begin with, "Have you told your mother you are pregnant?" If Juana's mother is going to be involved in her pregnancy, it would also be important to have her come along to the prenatal visits. In terms of care for a new child, the grandmother's role may become more important in Juana's day-to-day activities. Important details of Juana's life, such as who will take care of the baby, the role of the grandmother, and her eligibility for publicly funded programs, are critical facts that will influence her health care needs and the availability of resources.

Because of universal screening recommendations during pregnancy, Juana consented to be tested for HIV. Her HIV test was positive, and her viral load was very high, indicating active HIV disease. Her HIV diagnosis is discussed and appropriate retroviral treatment is begun. She returns by herself for her 6-month prenatal visit, and the pregnancy is progressing well without other complications. Juana did tell her mother, who is 45 years old, that she is pregnant, and her mother is now looking forward to being a grandparent. However, Juana decided not to share her HIV diagnosis and treatment details with her because of

> *her mother's low opinion of people who have AIDS. Her mother has said, "I know parents of too many drug users and promiscuous children who have contracted AIDS. Those bad parents are responsible for their children's risky behaviors and I am quite proud of my only daughter, who has remained sensible and disease-free." Juana states jokingly, "I know she would throw me out onto the street if she ever found out I was HIV-positive."*

3 If Juana has HIV, does that mean her newborn baby will be born HIV-positive?

Not necessarily. Current treatment options for HIV-positive, pregnant patients vary and depend on how far along the woman is in the pregnancy. Asymptomatic women in the first trimester of pregnancy may consider delaying treatment until after 10 to 12 weeks. [After the first trimester, minimum treatment should include azidothymidine (AZT)]. Other factors, such as CD4 count, viral load, and drug resistance, should be considered to determine the best treatment option for an individual patient. Although preliminary teratogenicity data are reassuring, the use of other anti-HIV medications in pregnancy must be carefully monitored due to the limited knowledge about the safety profile of these drugs for the mother and fetus.

Treatment during labor and delivery is recommended, as the major risk for transmission of HIV from mother to neonate occurs around this time. Currently, the most common course of therapy is the three-part AZT regimen. It includes AZT (100 mg five times per day, 200 mg three times per day, or 300 mg two times per day) starting at 14 to 34 weeks, intravenous AZT during parturition, and treatment of the baby for 6 weeks with oral AZT. Although the exact mechanisms of vertical transmission are unknown, treating the mother and baby in this manner reduces the transmission rate to 5–8%. (Many women continue their other anti-HIV medications during labor and should discuss this with their providers.)

4 What are the concerns and fears Juana may have regarding her diagnosis? Is it acceptable for Juana to exercise autonomy by withholding information from her mother?

Although a diagnosis of HIV infection or AIDS may not carry a stigma for Juana and young people her age, it may still mean great social stigma for those of the generation of Juana's mother. Juana's joking assertion that her mother would throw her out was a reflection of a deeper and certainly understandable fear about her mother's possible reaction and the loss of her support and affection. However, despite Juana's fears about the potential reaction of her mother, it would be important for Juana to consider initiating a conversation with her mother about these issues since it is very likely that Mrs. Cabon will discover that Juana is taking medications for HIV infection. As a prelude to this conversation with her mother, it would be useful for the physicians to have a discussion with Juana pertaining to her beliefs about the HIV illness and its treatment. In addition, helping patients disclose their HIV status is usually a process and having Juana connected with a multidisciplinary team experienced in care of HIV-positive patients may increase her support and resources.

Ultimately, as an adult, Juana clearly has the legal right to make medical decisions regarding herself and her unborn child without informing her mother. A patient decision such as this can illicit reactions of anger and frustration in the physicians. In managing these emotions, it is important for the caregivers to recognize any personal biases they might have regarding HIV-positive patients and caring for an unwed mother.

> *Although Juana was compliant with her treatment regimen and had no undue adverse effects from the medication, her viral load remained very high. As she approached her ninth month of pregnancy, Dr. Graham informed Juana that, with a high viral load, the baby's risk of HIV infection would be decreased if a cesarian section were performed. Juana responded, "I want to do whatever is best for the baby, but I don't want to be cut. I also don't want the C-section because, if I have it, my mother might figure out I am HIV-positive." After some further conversation with Dr. Graham, Juana says, "I might consider the C-section if you promise to tell my mom there is some other reason for the C-section. The baby is too big or something like that." The obstetrics team meets to discuss Juana's case.*

5   Is the obstetrics team being asked to lie? Is the obstetrician's recommendation for C-section in the best interest of Juana? Who is (or should be) the patient in this case?

The physicians here are faced with sorting through an ethically complex situation in which there is apparent conflict between several professional and legal obligations. On one hand, Juana has the right to make her own medical decisions (autonomy) and the expectation that her conversations with the physicians are privileged and confidential (confidentiality). However, the physicians are required to be truthful (veracity) and act in the best interest of the patient (beneficence). The issue of beneficence becomes even more challenging in that there are two patients (Juana and her baby) whose interests need to be attended to, but which may conflict.

In terms of disclosure to the mother, the legal issue is straightforward. Federal regulations [i.e. those based on the Health Insurance Portability and Accountability Act (HIPPA] are in place to insure the privacy and security of patient information. These regulations prohibit the release of patient information without the consent of the patient (although they are not meant to be a barrier to emergent or appropriate care). Consequently, in this case, Mrs. Caban is not the patient and the patient's wishes for confidentiality should be respected. However, given the lack of a social network and support beyond her mother, it might be in Juana's best interest, and that of her baby, to inform her mother and bring her fully into the circle of care. Physicians are expected to be honest, truthful, transparent, and open, and thus to lie to the mother about the indication for the cesarean would violate a core physician value. But, if this would enable Juana to consent to the surgery, and thus give the baby the opportunity to have the best outcome, might this be one of those rare instances when deception by the physician would be acceptable?

A case such as this is filled with subtleties and nuances, and the context is always important. However, if Juana does continue to decline a cesarean section, then the most ethically defensible approach is to accept her decision and use available medical therapy to prevent transmission of HIV to the infant; make appropriate, good faith efforts to protect her privacy; and decline to be willfully or knowingly deceptive.

6   What response might you make to Juana's request if you were the obstetrician or PCP?

After clarifying the issues among themselves, the care team should continue to engage Juana in supportive, respectful, and patient discussion about her concerns and fears, ensuring that the physician recommendations have been presented in a clear and understandable matter. Offering to have Juana speak to her mother in the office, with the physician present, may provide a level of safety and comfort that will enable her to overcome her fears. Enlisting the assistance and advice of trained clinicians experienced in the care of HIV-positive patients may also be helpful. Although the physicians may disagree, ultimately the decision to have the cesarean section, or disclose her diagnosis, is Juana's. She, however, should understand that, although every effort will be made to maintain the privacy of her diagnosis, the staff will not allow itself to be put in position where they will be made to lie. Instead, if asked directly about the reason for the cesarean section, the care team will decline to answer the question and direct the question to Juana.

References: Case 18

ACOG Committee Opinion. Prenatal and Perinatal Human Immunodeficiency Virus Testing: Expanded Recommendations, Number 304, November 2004.

ACOG Committee Opinion. Scheduled Cesarean Delivery and the Prevention of Vertical Transmission of HIV Infection, Number 234, May 2000.

DaSilva C.H., Cunta R.L., Tonaco R.B. Not telling the truth in the patient-physician relationship. *Bioethics* 2003;17:417–24.

Gadow S. Truth: treatment of choice, scarce resource, or patients' right? *J Fam Pract* 1981;13:857–60.

HIV During Pregnancy, Labor and Delivery, and After Birth, U.S. Department of Health and Human Services, 2006.

Hochhauser M. Therapeutic misconception and "recruiting doublespeak" in the informed consent process. *IRB* 2002;24:11–12.

Hutchings D. Communicating with metaphor: a dance with many veils. *Am J Palliat Care* 1998;15:282–4.

Levine R.J. Consent to incomplete disclosure as an alternative to deception: case study. *IRB* 1982;4:9–11.

Maternal therapy among infants in the women and infants transmission study. *J Acquir Immune Defic Syndr* 2007;44(3):299–305.

Newell M.L., Huang S., Fiore S., et al. For the PSCTG 316 Study Team: Characteristics and management of HIV-1-infected pregnant women enrolled in a randomized trial: differences between Europe and the USA. *BMC Infect Dis* 2007;7:60.

Public Health Service Task Force Recommendations for Use of Antiretroviral Drugs in Pregnant HIV-Infected Women for Maternal Health and Interventions to Reduce Perinatal HIV Transmission in the United States, November 2007.

Satcher D., Pamies R.J. Case studies. In *Multicultural Medicine and Health Disparities*. McGraw-Hill Companies, Columbus, 2006, pp 361–8.

Simpson D.E., Yindra K.J., Towne J.B., Rosenfeld P.S. Medical students' perceptions of cheating. *Acad Med* 1989;64:221–2.

Tucker A.G. Truth-telling in clinical practice and the arguments for and against: a review of the literature. *Nurs Ethics* 2004;11:500–13.

Watts D.H. Effect of pregnancy. *J Acquir Immune Defic Syndr* 2005;38(1):S36–8.

Watts D.H. Treating HIV during pregnancy: an update on safety issues. *Drug Saf* 2006;29(6):467–90.

Watts DH. Teratogenicity risk of antiretroviral therapy in pregnancy. *Curr HIV/AIDS Repr* 2007;4(3):135–40.

Watts D.H., Daner L., Handelsman E., et al. Assessment of birth defects according to maternal therapy among infants in the women and infants transmission study. *J Acquir Immune Defic Syndr* 2007;44(3):299–305.

CASE 19

Alice Gregory

A 71-year-old African American woman with aortic stenosis

Susan E. Wiegers, MD and Horace DeLisser, MD

University of Pennsylvania School of Medicine, Philadelphia, PA, USA

Educational Objectives

- Describe the potential impact of patient bias or prejudice on the patient–physician relationship.
- Practice correct techniques for responding to offensive or inappropriate comments or questions by patients.
- List strategies and boundaries for negotiating patient preferences.

TACCT Domains: 1, 3, 4, 6

Case Summary, Questions and Answers

Mrs. Gregory is a 71-year-old African American woman who came to the cardiology clinic for evaluation of aortic stenosis, which was detected on an echocardiogram (ECG) after her primary care provider (PCP) noted a loud systolic murmur. She was scheduled to see a first-year fellow, Dr. Dinh Nueyang, a Vietnamese American physician, whose parents were refugees from South East Asia, but who was born and raised in Southern California. Upon entering the room and extending his hand to introduce himself, Mrs. Gregory immediately asked him, "Do you speak good English?" Dr. Nueyang replied angrily, "Of course I speak English well! I don't know why you would even ask."

Achieving Cultural Competency: A case-based approach to training health professionals,
1st edition. Edited by L Hark, H DeLisser. © 2009 Blackwell Publishing,
ISBN: 9781405180726.

1   Why might Mrs. Gregory have asked this question?

This encounter could merely be a clumsy or awkward remark from an anxious patient who may be frustrated over past experiences with foreign medical doctors where it had been difficult to understand the physician. The question may also be a reflection of a cultural stereotype, but asked without any real malice or ill will or it could in fact be an expression of a more malignant prejudice or bias. Just as physician bias may enter and influence the doctor–patient relationship, past experiences and prejudices of patients may also impact the relationship.

Foreign (International) Medical Graduates

Foreign medical graduates (FMGs) constitute a quarter of all physicians in the United States and account for 27% of the country's residents and fellows. Were it not for FMGs, many residency-training positions in pediatrics, anesthesiology, psychiatry, and family medicine would be otherwise vacant. Further, because the United States is currently experiencing a physician shortage, the United States will continue to rely heavily on FMGs to meet this shortfall, especially in the areas of primary care and in underserved populations and regions.

As noted by McMahon (2004), "both physicians and their patients can find language barriers frustrating. Despite the requirement of the Educational Commission for Foreign Medical Graduates (ECFMG) for the demonstration of competence in English, only physicians with previous immersion among English speakers can reach the level of fluency that is typically required for discussions about medical decisions. When patients report what may be genuine problems with doctor–patient communication, their complaints can be interpreted, rightly or wrongly, as evidence of intolerance or racism and can strike a further blow to the self-esteem of immigrants who are already struggling against suspicion."

Dr. Nueyang subsequently spent 5 minutes obtaining a history and completing his examination. He then left the room to discuss his evaluation with Dr. Laura Brown, his supervising attending. He informed Dr. Brown that the patient was a poor historian, but would likely need surgery for aortic stenosis. When Dr. Brown asked him whether Mrs. Gregory knew she might need surgery, Dr. Nueyang replied, "No I did not discuss surgery with her. You will need to talk to her about that."

2   Why might Dr. Nueyang have been angered or hurt by Mrs. Gregory's question?

Physicians of Asian ancestry, even those born in the U.S., report that it is not uncommon for patients to ask questions or make comments that reflect suspicions about their skill or competence as physicians because they are Asian. For Dr. Nueyang, who has excelled academically, this question (which he has encountered on several previous occasions), and its possible implications with respect to his competence, is a source of anger for him. In a later conversation with Dr. Brown, Dr. Nueyang admitted, "It hurt me that an African American woman would say something like that. You would think she would be more sensitive."

3   How should Dr. Nueyang have responded to Mrs. Gregory's questions?

The goal is to respond to patients in a way that is honest and authentic, yet respectful and tactful, in order to ultimately create a therapeutic relationship with the patient. It is important for each physician to have an awareness of the comments or behaviors that patients might say or do that trigger anger or other emotions. When a button has been pushed, the physician needs to first recognize the emotion and then maintain control. Sometimes it makes sense to simply ignore or overlook such a comment and move on with the patient encounter. (Now is not the right time; or this battle is not worth fighting.) *"Sure, I speak English. I was born in the U.S. And now I would like to ask you a few questions to see how I can help you to feel better."* And there will be (rare) instances where the emotion is so strong and distracting, that the physician will need to leave the room in order to collect him/herself or find some one else to complete the examination. The inability of a physician to be self-aware and modulate his or her reactions is likely to influence the development of rapport.

However, because of the importance of open and honest communication between the patient and the physician, in most instances, the physician should initiate a respectful discussion with the patient about the inappropriate or offensive question or comment. Such a conversation allows the physician to channel his/her anger as well as define the boundaries of the relationship. By responding without harshness, it prevents a defensive counter-reaction from the patient. *"Actually my English is quite good. I am surprised that you would ask me something like that. Please share with me what prompted you to ask this kind of question."*

> Upon entering the exam room with Dr. Nueyang, Dr. Brown immediately recognizes that Mrs. Gregory is angry, as she is sitting with her arms crossed and has an obvious look of disgust. Dr. Brown introduces herself and asks Mrs. Gregory how she was doing. Turning toward Dr. Nueyang, Mrs. Gregory angrily says, "I asked him a question that made him mad. But I am paying him and I am allowed to ask him any question I want."
>
> Dr. Brown responds, "Yes sure, you can ask him any questions, but I don't think you made him mad, because he did not tell me that you made him mad. He, in fact, described you as pleasant." Dr. Brown notices that Dr. Nueyang is visibly angry, frowning, gritting his teeth and says, "You are right, he looks angry. What did you ask him?"
>
> And Mrs. Gregory says, "I asked him if he spoke English."
>
> Laughing, Dr. Brown replies, "Of course he speaks English. He was born in the United States. I have known him for 4 years and he speaks perfect English. He is also fluent in Vietnamese. Did you have trouble understanding him?"
>
> "No, but I don't care that he speaks Vietnamese, only English," replies Mrs. Gregory. "Besides, I am not comfortable with him. I don't want him to be my doctor. I want someone else."

4 Should the patient's request be honored, particularly if it might reflect a bias or prejudice on the part of the patient?

Not surprisingly, patients, across a range of racial and ethnic groups, when asked to choose a physician, will tend to select a physician who appears to be from their racial or ethnic group. Possible reasons for this include the following:

- a belief that a physician from one's own racial or ethnic background can better understand and attend to specific health concerns;
- a desire to avoid a racist physician and racism.

In this situation, the decision is further complicated by the fact that Dr. Nueyang displayed anger toward the patient. Such behavior, however justifiable in his eyes, may have made this situation unredeemable and it might be best to honor this patient's request.

It has been proposed that having a physician of the same race/ethnicity as that of the patient may promote more effective communication, greater trust of the physician, and facilitate better mutual understanding of the patient's health concerns, behaviors, and expectations. Research suggests that race/ethnicity concordance in the patient–physician relationship is associated with greater utilization and quality of primary and specialty care, improved partnership in decision making, and greater satisfaction with care. It should be noted, however, that racial and ethnic concordance between the patient and the physician is not always associated with improved outcomes or better patient care.

Ultimately, our health care system gives patients the right to choose their health care providers. There are, however, values we do want to protect and promote, such as nondiscriminatory care. Although it is appropriate to make reasonable accommodations for the desires and comfort of the patient, encouragement should not be given to patient behaviors that undermine these core values. In fact, physician role modeling of inclusivity and respect of others (such as trainees who may be of a different gender or ethnicity) is important in enabling patients to effectively navigate through the health care system. The hard questions include:

- What constitutes a reasonable accommodation?
- How far should we go in endorsing the preferences of patients?

Some make a distinction between choosing *for* versus choosing *against* someone. However, is it permissible to select a gynecologist because the physician is a woman, or to choose a black internist because the patient would be more comfortable with an African American doctor, but wrong to decline to see the Muslim neurologist because the Christian patient believes he could relate better to another Christian?

References: Case 19

Bach P.B., Pham H.H., Schrag D., Tate R.C., Hargraves J.L. Primary care physicians who treat blacks and whites. *N Engl J Med* 2004;351:575–84.

Boulet J.R., Norcini J.J., Whelan G.P., Hallock J.A., Seeling S.S. The international medical graduate pipeline: recent trends in certification and residency training. *Health Aff* 2006;25:469–77.

Chilton J.A., Gor B.J., Hajek R.A., Jones L.A. Cervical cancer among Vietnamese women: efforts to define the problem among Houston's population. *Gynecol Oncol* 2005;99(3):S203–6 (suppl 1).

Faggiano P., Antonini-Canterin F., Baldessin F., Lorusso R., D'Aloia A., Cas L.D. Epidemiology and cardiovascular risk factors of aortic stenosis. *Cardiovasc Ultrasound* 2006;4:27.

Fiscella K., Frankel R. Overcoming cultural barriers: international medical graduates in the United States. *JAMA* 2000;283:1751.

Gerbert B., Berg-Smith S., Mancuso M., et al. Video study of physician selection: preferences in the face of diversity. *J Fam Pract* 2003;52:552–9.

Lew A.A., Moskowitz J.M., Ngo L., et al. Effect of provider status on preventive screening among Korean-American women in Alameda County, California. *Prev Med* 2003;36:141–9.

McMahon G.T. Coming to America: international medical graduates in the United States. *N Engl J Med* 2004;350:2435–7.

O'Brien K.D. Pathogenesis of calcific aortic valve disease: a disease process comes of age (and a good deal more). *Arterioscler Thromb Vasc Biol* 2006;26:1721–8.

Otto C.M. Valvular aortic stenosis: disease severity and timing of intervention. *J Am Coll Cardiol* 2006;47:2141–51.

Stevens G.D., Mistry R., Zuckerman B., Halfon N. The parent-provider relationship: does race/ethnicity concordance or discordance influence parent reports of the receipt of high quality basic pediatric preventive services? *J Urban Health* 2005;82:560–74.

Tu S.P., Yasui Y., Kuniyuki A., Schwartz S.M., Jackson J.C., Taylor V.M. Breast cancer screening: stages of adoption among Cambodian American women. *Cancer Detect Prev* 2002;26:33–41.

Verghese A. Resident redux. *Ann Intern Med* 2004;140:1034–6.

Whelan G. High-stakes medical performance testing: the Clinical Skills Assessment program. *JAMA* 2000;283:1748.

Whelan G.P., Gary N.E., Kostis J., Boulet J.R., Hallock J.A. The changing pool of international medical graduates seeking certification training in US graduate medical education programs. *JAMA* 2002;288:1079–84.

Yee B.W.K. Health and Healthcare of Southeast Asian American Elders: Vietnamese, Cambodian, Hmong, and Laotian elders. Available at: http://www.stanford.edu/group/ethnoger/southeasian.html.

CASE 20

Sunil Guha

A 32-year-old South Asian Indian man with metabolic syndrome

Fran Burke, MS, RD,[1] *and Lisa Hark, PhD, RD*[2]

[1] University of Pennsylvania School of Medicine, Philadelphia, PA, USA
[2] Jefferson Medical College, Philadelphia, PA, USA

Educational Objectives

- Identify risk factors for coronary heart disease specific for the Asian Indian population.
- Describe how acculturation to a Western society may affect the lifestyle of the Asian Indian migrant.
- Discuss why it is important to understand how cultural and ethnic factors play a role in treatment recommendations.
- Propose a nutrition and physical activity plan for an Asian Indian patient at risk of coronary heart disease.

TACCT Domains: 1, 2, 4

Case Summary, Questions and Answers

Sunil Guha is a 32-year-old Asian Indian man who is seen in the Preventive Cardiology Clinic for a consultation. He has referred himself because he is concerned about his family history of premature heart disease (his father had his first myocardial infarction at 45), and he is seeking ways in which he can prevent this from happening to him. He has been living in the U.S. for the past 11 years since he came over for college. He is an engineer, recently married, and is planning to start a family in the near future. His parents still live in India, and he visits them a few times a

Achieving Cultural Competency: A case-based approach to training health professionals,
1st edition. Edited by L Hark, H DeLisser. © 2009 Blackwell Publishing,
ISBN: 9781405180726.

year. He brings his lab results with him to the visit, which he obtained while visiting his primary care physician (PCP) a few months ago. He states that he does not want to take medication and prefers to focus on changing his diet and lifestyle. Mr. Guha's results are as follows:

1 Is Mr. Guha at higher risk of heart disease compared with the general population, and how does his ethnic background affect his risk?

Yes, Mr. Guha is at greater risk for coronary heart disease (CHD) because he has several cardiac risk factors, including a family history of premature heart disease and metabolic syndrome. Mr. Guha is diagnosed with metabolic syndrome because he meets three of the four criteria: increased waist circumference (WC), borderline elevated blood pressure, elevated blood sugar, and elevated triglyceride levels (shown in Table 20.2).

Asian Indians are at higher risk for CHD, which occurs about 5 to 10 years earlier than in other populations. The increased risk appears to be due to the higher rates of metabolic syndrome, insulin resistance, and diabetes. Healthy, normal weight Asian Indians are more likely to have insulin resistance compared with age- and BMI-matched whites. Furthermore, insulin resistance in Asian Indians manifests at an earlier age. Conventional criteria from the Adult Treatment Panel (ATP) III underestimates the prevalence of metabolic syndrome by 25% to 50% in Asian Indians,

Table 20.1 Mr. Guha's Lab Results

	Visit 1	Desirable
Blood pressure	135/85 mm Hg	<130/80
Fasting blood glucose	100 mg/dL	<99
Fasting triglyceride	210 mg/dL	<150
HDL-C	40 mg/dL	>40
LDL-C (direct measure)	116 mg/dL	<130
Total cholesterol	190 mg/dL	<200
Height	5'6"	
Weight	167 lbs	
Body Mass Index (BMI)	27	<25
Waist circumference (WC)	36"	<35*

*based on International Diabetes Foundation definition, http://www.idf.org.

Table 20.2 Diagnosing Metabolic Syndrome:
three or more of the five criteria

Abdominal obesity	Waist circumference
	Men >40 inches
	Women >35 inches
Pre-Hypertension	BP ≥130/≥85 mm Hg
Glucose intolerance	FBG ≥110 mg/dL
High triglycerides	≥150 mg/dL
Low HDL-C	Men <40 mg/dL
	Women <50 mg/dL

Source: Adult Treatment Panel (ATP) III Guidelines,
NCEP 2001 Report.

because this ethnic group develops metabolic abnormalities at a lower BMI and WC than other ethnic groups. Therefore, several national and international organizations have recommended using the International Diabetes Federation (IDF) definition, which has developed ethnic- and gender-specific criteria using WC criteria for central obesity as a mandatory component (Table 20.3).

Most studies indicate that the average BMI of Asian Indians increases with urbanization and migration but is still less than that seen in whites, Mexican Americans, and blacks. Mr. Guha's BMI is 27 inches and his WC is 36 inches. He meets the IDF criteria for increased WC, in addition to having an elevated blood pressure and triglyceride level at his first visit. Therefore, he should be treated with aggressive lifestyle management.

Table 20.3 Ethnic and gender WC criteria for central obesity

	Men (inches)	Women (inches)
European		
Sub-Sahara Africa	>37	>32
Middle eastern		
South Asian		
South/Central American	>35	>32
Japanese		
Chinese		

Source: International Diabetes Federation.

2   What other laboratory values would be helpful in determining treatment recommendations for this patient?

In addition to a comprehensive metabolic and lipid panel, Mr. Guha should also be tested for lipoprotein [Lp(a)] and apolipoprotein B. Asian Indians often present with a dyslipidemia that is characterized by high serum levels of apolipoprotein B, Lp(a), and triglycerides and low levels of apolipoprotein A1 and high-density lipoprotein cholesterol (HDL-C). An elevated apolipoprotein B level is a stronger risk factor for CAD than low-density lipoprotein cholesterol (LDL-C) and is found in one-third of Asian Indians.

Several studies report a strong association between Lp(a) levels and CHD risk. Lp(a) is a modified form of LDL-C. It represents a class of LDL-C particles that have apolipoprotein B-100 linked to apolipoprotein A. Lp(a) is structurally similar to plasminogen but has no thrombolytic activity. Excess Lp(a) may promote atherosclerosis by increasing LDL oxidation and smooth muscle cell proliferation and by impairing endothelium-dependent vasodilation. Plasma Lp(a) levels are determined primarily by genetic factors that regulate production by the liver. Screening for Lp(a) is recommended for patients with a strong family history of premature CHD, as in Mr. Guha's case. Lp(a) measurement is useful for identifying high-risk individuals and families who may be at higher risk than what might be suggested by mildly elevated total or LDL-C levels. These patients may benefit from earlier pharmacotherapy in conjunction with diet and lifestyle changes.

The optimal level of Lp(a) should be less than 20 mg/dL. Research shows that the risk of CAD is two- to fourfold higher when the levels of Lp(a) are above 30 to 40 mg/dL. This risk also increases when an Lp(a) level greater than 50 mg/dL is accompanied by elevated cholesterol levels. Recent studies have indicated that CAD risk is much greater when elevated Lp(a) levels are accompanied by low HDL-C versus high LDL-C levels.

Mr. Guha's Lp(a) results are 61 mg/dL and aggressive therapy is warranted, but he states that he does not want to take medication and prefers to focus on changing his diet and lifestyle. He is referred to a registered dietitian who determines that he is a vegetarian and his diet includes white rice, legumes, and whole milk dairy products. He has been eating a combination of American and Indian foods since he began living in the United States 11 years ago. He states that he tries to watch what he eats and only eats one meal per day with no snacks.

3 How does Mr. Guha's ethnic background affect his dietary habits and lifestyle?

Nutrition interventions for the prevention and treatment of CAD need to be compatible with an individual's cultural values and beliefs. Developing nutrition interventions that target people from diverse backgrounds presents a variety of challenges. Health professionals must recognize the importance of specific foods within cultures and of ethnosocial influences on food choices. However, generalizations about food patterns should not be made solely on the basis of race, ethnicity, or geographic origin because food-choice diversity is common within all cultural and racial groups. The U.S. is a melting pot of cultures. Interventions are most effective when focused on each individual's unique dietary history and background, without making assumptions about food habits on the basis of cultural or racial identity. Factors such as where you live may influence the availability of ethnic foods, and issues of acculturation play a huge role in the food selection of all people.

Asian Indians often follow a vegetarian diet for both cultural and religious reasons. Rice and wheat are staples of the Indian diet, whereas fruit and vegetable intakes are low. Many vegetarian foods and baked goods are prepared with coconut and palm oils, butter, ghee (clarified butter), vanaspathi (hydrogenated fat), and coconut milk, all of which are very high in saturated and trans fats.

It is important to question Mr. Guha about the types of fats that he and his family use when preparing Indian dishes at home. His saturated fat intake should be less than 7% of his total calorie intake. Asian Indians in India consume relatively more carbohydrates (~60% to 67% of energy intake) compared with Asian Indians living in the U.S. (~56% to 58% of energy intake). High carbohydrate intake is associated with elevated triglyceride levels. Low dietary intake and low plasma levels of omega-3 fatty acids in Asian Indians have been reported in several studies.

Asian Indians have been shown to be less physically active compared with other ethnic groups. It is culturally unacceptable for Muslin women to participate in leisure time physical activity. Mr. Guha currently leads a very sedentary lifestyle. Sedentary Asian Indians are more likely to have higher BMI values, triglyceride levels, and blood pressure. Physical activity patterns in Asian Indians warrant further investigation because a sedentary lifestyle could be an important risk factor for the insulin resistance seen in this population.

Whoever prepares meals for this family should be included in the counseling session with the dietitian.

The dietitian prescribes a low saturated fat diet and a regular exercise program, both of which are supported by the physician. Mr. Guha says he will return for follow-up in 3 months; however, he does not. He returns to the Preventive Cardiology Clinic 3 years later. His father died of heart disease the previous year. He also states that his mother, who has diabetes, has been living with his family since last year and now does most of the cooking. He reports that he has been very busy with work and his new 1-year-old baby and rarely finds time to exercise.

---

4   What is the best approach to take with this patient who has not followed up as recommended?

Initially patients may express the desire to change lifestyle habits and appear motivated to improve their overall health but may find it challenging to make permanent dietary changes. When patients do not return for their follow-up visit, it typically means that they have not followed the medical nutrition prescription that was outlined for them.

From a gender perspective, Mr. Guha may follow a sex role belief that women cook and men eat, therefore imparting him with an adopted powerlessness about food that his mother and wife prepare. Being aware of this would be important in developing an effective behavior charge program for Mr. Guha.

Bringing patients back frequently for follow-up visits and asking them to complete food and activity records is a good behavioral tool to keep patients on track. The best way to discuss these issues with Mr. Guha is to explain where he is in terms of his CHD risk, where he needs to be to lower his risk, and how we can achieve this together. This provides a supportive, nonjudgmental approach. It is important to inform Mr. Guha that you appreciate him returning for follow-up, rather than confronting him with your disappointment that he has not come back for 3 years.

Vital signs and labs are obtained (see Table 20.4). Mr. Guha returns 1 week later to discuss his lab results.

Table 20.4 Mr. Guha's lab results

	Visit 1:	Visit 2: (3 years later)
Blood pressure	135/85 mm Hg	150/86 mm Hg
Fasting blood glucose	100 mg/dL	122 mg/dL
Fasting triglyceride	210 mg/dL	250 mg/dL
HDL-C	40 mg/dL	35 mg/dL
LDL-C	116 mg/dL	152 mg/dL
Total cholesterol	190 mg/dL	230 mg/dL
Height	5'6"	5'6"
Weight	167 lbs	182 lbs
BMI (kg/m^2)	27	29
WC	36"	39"
Lp(a)	61	68

5   What is the most appropriate next step in the management of this patient?

At this point, it is important to express concern about Mr. Guha's increased weight as well as the significant increase in many of his lab values. Focus on the nonweight goals when counseling Mr. Guha. He should understand that he now meets all five of the ATP III criteria for metabolic syndrome and, because of his strong family history for premature CHD, he is at high risk for developing heart disease. In addition, because his mother has diabetes and his blood sugar is now elevated, he is also at risk of developing diabetes. Mr. Guha should therefore be aggressively treated with diet, exercise, and medication(s) to reduce his risk of heart disease and diabetes. Mr. Guha's diet should be low in saturated and trans fats and restricted in total calories to achieve weight loss. Recommend that he substitute lower fat dairy products for those that are high in saturated fat, such as cheese and whole milk yogurt. The patient needs to increase his total and soluble fiber intake by substituting whole grain starches for the white bread and white rice he consumes daily.

The predominant cooking oil used in food preparation should be high in monounsaturated fat, such as olive or canola oil. In addition, Mr. Guha and his mom should be counseled to avoid frying, or use a limited amount of oil to sauté or stir fry foods, as oils are calorically dense, supplying 135 calories per tablespoon. Mr. Guha should be encouraged to increase his intake of fresh fruits and vegetables, which will help increase his fiber intake, decrease the energy density of his diet, and help him better manage his weight. Finally,

Mr. Guha should be counseled to avoid drinking sugar-sweetened beverages, such as regular soda or fruit juice. These beverages, which provide refined sugars, contribute to increased calories and elevated triglyceride and glucose levels. Finally, Mr. Guha is recommended to begin a physical activity program three to four times a week for at least 30 minutes, which will aid in weight control and may help to improve HDL-C levels.

The physician starts Mr. Guha on several medications in addition to recommending lifestyle changes, which include an aspirin, anti-hypertensive agent, and an HMG CoA reductase inhibitor. ATP III details the means of assessing CHD risk and outlining LDL target goals, which for Mr. Guha, is less than 100 mg/dL. A follow-up appointment with the physician and registered dietitian is scheduled for 6 weeks to monitor changes in serum lipids, glucose, blood pressure, and weight and reassess medications.

6   What factors have contributed to the change in Mr. Guha's risk factor profile?

By helping Mr. Guha reassess his life and identify factors that have contributed to his overall health, he is more likely to come to terms with his current health problems and begin to make lifestyle changes to prevent future events. It is very important that Mr. Guha maintain his cultural identity, especially related to his food intake and physical activity pattern, by providing culturally appropriate recommendations targeted to Asian Indian patients. These are the factors in Mr. Guha's life:

Lifestyle: He has a full-time job and a new baby and states that he is very, very busy and does not have time to exercise. Mr. Guha would greatly benefit from a regular exercise program, so discussing how he can work in time to exercise or make exercise part of his everyday life is critical. Write him an exercise prescription and discuss his schedule and activities he enjoys. Suggest he purchase a pedometer to help quantify his activity, and discuss activities he enjoyed when he was more active. Encourage reducing sedentary activities, such as limiting television and taking stairs instead of elevators.

Stress: The death of his father and the stress at work have placed much pressure on Mr. Guha, which has caused him to eat more, exercise less, and avoid focusing on his own health. Ask him if he has ever paid attention to stress reduction and if he would be willing to try meditation, yoga, and massage therapy, as some may fit into his cultural belief systems.

Preparation of the family meals: Now that Mr. Guha's mother is living with his family on a full-time basis, she is taking care of their child and cooking all their meals. As a result, he states that he has gained

Table 20.5 Healthier versions of traditional Asian Indian cuisine

Traditional food	Healthier way of eating
Meat, poultry, fish, and eggs fried in ghee, butter, coconut oil, palm kernel oil, or hydrogenated fats and oils.	Bake, roast, broil, grill, or oven-fry. Remove skin from chicken before eating. Fry with canola, olive, or corn oil instead. Limit to 1/4 cup of oil.
Legumes and vegetables prepared with oil, butter, cream yogurt to enhance flavor.	Use almond paste or nonfat yogurt in place of cream and butter. Season with onion, garlic, spices, or low-sodium chicken broth to enhance flavor.
Rice (white) dishes or wheat (refined) preparations deep fried or prepared with large amounts of ghee, butter, and hydrogenated fats (vanaspati) containing trans fatty acids.	Use brown rice and whole grain wheat. Boil or bake instead of frying. Fry with canola, olive, or corn oil or trans-free margarine instead of solid or hydrogenated fat. Limit to 1/4 cup of oil.
Whole milk/cheese/cream/yogurt used to prepare rice dishes, vegetables, desserts, and shakes. Yogurt cheese (panir) prepared with whole milk.	Use low-fat or nonfat milk, milk powder, cheese, cream, yogurt, buttermilk, or soymilk instead.
Omelettes and desserts prepared with egg yolks.	Substitute egg yolks with egg whites.
Snacks such as fried legumes "bhel."	Snack on fruits, rice cakes, and puddings made with low-fat milk instead. Use oat and whole wheat cereal to prepare savory snacks.
Salt used to enhance flavor.	Use herbs (e.g. cilantro, mint) or spices (e.g. cumin, black pepper, cardamom, cinnamon) or flaxseed powder to enhance flavor.

Source: Gans, K., Karmally W. Multicultural nutrition strategies: Asian-Indians. In: Carson J.S., Burke F.M., Hark L.A., eds. *Cardiovascular Nutrition: Disease Management and Prevention.* American Dietetic Association, Chicago, 2004.

15 pounds in the past few years. Mr. Guha's BMI is 29, combined with an increased WC of 39 inches, significantly increases his risk of CHD. To help improve adherence, include his mother and wife as part of the conversation with the registered dietitian to ensure that she can still prepare and enjoy a healthier Indian cuisine. Refer to Table 20.4 for healthier versions of traditional Asian cuisine.

References: Case 20

Enas E.A., Chacko V., Pazhoor S.G., Chennikkara H., Devarapalli H.P. Dyslipidemia in South Asian patients. *Curr Atheroscler Rep* 2007;9(5):367–74.

Expert Panel on Detection, Evaluation, and Treatment of High Blood Cholesterol in Adults. Executive summary of the third report of the national cholesterol education program (NCEP) expert panel on detection, evaluation, and treatment of high blood cholesterol in adults (Adult Treatment Panel III). *JAMA* 2001;285:2486–97.

Gans K., Karmally W. Multicultural nutrition strategies. In: Carson J.S., Burke F.M, Hark L.A., eds.*Cardiovascular Nutrition: Disease Management and Prevention*. American Dietetic Association, Chicago, 2004.

Gupta R., Joshi P., Mohan V., Reddy K.S., Yusuf S. Epidemiology and causation of coronary heart disease and stroke in India. *Heart* 2008;94:16–26.

Hoogeveen R.C., Gambhir J.K., Gambhir D.S. Evaluation of Lp(a) and other independent risk factors for CHD in Asian-Indians and their USA counterparts. *J Lipid Res* 2001;42:631–8.

Joshi P., Islam S., Pais P., et al. Risk factors for early myocardial infarction in South Asians compared with individuals in other countries. *JAMA* 2007;297:286–94.

Minority Women's Health. Available at: http://www.4woman.gov.

Misra A., Vikram N.K. Insulin resistance syndrome (metabolic syndrome) and obesity in Asian-Indians:evidence and implications. *Nutrition* 2004; 20:482–91.

Rajeshwari R., Nicklas T.A., Pownall H.J., Berenson G.S. Cardiovascular diseases-a major health risk in Asian-Indians. *Nutr Res* 2005;25:515–33.

von Eckardstein A., Schulte H., Cullen P. Lipoprotein(a) further increases the risk of coronary events in men with high global cardiovascular risk. *J Am Coll Cardiol* 2001;37:434–9.

CASE 21

Pepper Hawthorne

A 19-year-old Caucasian woman with a stroke

Scott Kasner, MD
University of Pennsylvania School of Medicine, Philadelphia, PA, USA

Educational Objectives

- Explain how a young woman's symptoms might be perceived as hysterical or psychogenic, particularly when there is little objective evidence of active disease.
- Assess how assumptions that might be made about patients based on their appearance and/or behavior, even if not directly relevant to their diagnosis may impact their access to care.
- Analyze how communication between health care personnel and patients may be distorted by erroneous perceptions.

TACCT Domains: 1, 3, 4, 6

Case Summary, Questions and Answers

Pepper Hawthorne is a 19-year-old college sophomore who developed sudden weakness and numbness of her left arm, and then the left side of her body, while studying for her final exams. Apart from endometriosis, for which she had recently undergone minor surgery, Ms. Hawthorne is otherwise healthy. She presented to the Emergency Department (ED)

Achieving Cultural Competency: A case-based approach to training health professionals,
1st edition. Edited by L Hark, H DeLisser. © 2009 Blackwell Publishing,
ISBN: 9781405180726.

1 hour after the onset of her symptoms and was immediately assessed by the triage nurse who noted that she was anxious, restless, and speaking rapidly. Suspecting that this was an anxiety attack, or malingering to get out of her exams, the nurse triaged Ms. Hawthorne as a nonurgent patient, saying to her, "Honey, have a seat and take some deep breaths. I think you are going to be just fine." Four hours later, she is called back into the treatment area to be seen by a physician. Although she was less anxious, she was still unable to move her left arm. Ms. Hawthorne becomes very tearful and emotional when asked by the physician about the duration of her "paralysis." He then asks, "Do you think you might be pregnant?"

She responded, "How could I be pregnant? I just had endometriosis surgery. Why won't anybody take me seriously?"

She is unable to move her left arm, but the physician suspects that this is volitional. Like the triage nurse, the ED physician is also suspicious that her symptoms are due to anxiety or stress and attempts to reassure her by saying, "I think you are going to be fine, but let's get a CT scan of your head to make sure everything is ok." He also orders a benzodiazapine.

1   What factors may have contributed to the nurse and the physician minimizing the significance of her symptoms?

Two interrelated factors, age and gender, coupled with Ms. Hawthorne's social situation may have contributed to minimization of her complaints. With respect to her age, the staff may have been influenced by the fact that stroke is much more common in middle-age and elderly patients. Stroke, however, in young adults is not exceptional; about 12% of first-time strokes occur in patients under age 45.

Physical findings suggestive of an acute stroke may also be found in patients with a conversion disorder, manifested by complaints of motor and/or sensory dysfunction without a neurological explanation. This disorder occurs in a younger age group (ages 10 to 50 years), predominately in women, and is often triggered by psychosocial stressors, all of which were present in this patient. Thus, entertaining the possibility of a conversion disorder was not inappropriate. However, gender stereotypes may have led the staff to conclude too quickly that the symptoms were "functional" in nature, due to either malingering or a conversion disorder.

Ellen Goudsmit, a clinical psychologist based in England who has worked extensively in the area of chronic fatigue syndrome, has written about what she calls the "psychologicalization of illness." She describes psychologicalization as "the emphasis on psychological factors where there is little or no evidence to justify it. It's a process where relevant findings are ignored or downplayed in favor of data from incomplete examinations, flawed research or anecdotal reports." In a clinical context, differential diagnoses may be dismissed prematurely, whereas psychological explanations are readily accepted. Psychologicalization does not refer to situations where there is sound evidence that psychological factors play a significant role or where all the arguments are discussed and the psychological explanations are deemed the most persuasive. Psychologicalization is a serious issue because it leads to misdiagnosis, inappropriate treatment, and unnecessary psychological distress. Moreover, it undermines the general population's confidence in orthodox medicine and reduces their trust in its practitioners.

With respect to women's health, there is good evidence that psychologicalization, although a feature of medicine in general, appears to disproportionately affect the care that women receive. The belief that psychological factors play a significant role in the complaints reported by women may explain in part why women may be evaluated less rigorously than men with similar complaints.

The patient's mother has arrived and is now in the examination room with her daughter. A CT scan of the head is obtained and shows early signs of a right frontal lobe infarction. After returning from the scan, Ms. Hawthorne is mildly lethargic from the sedative, and the ED physician now notes subtle drooping of the left side of her face. The stroke team is called to evaluate the patient, but she is no longer a candidate for acute thrombolytic therapy, as too much time has elapsed since the onset of her symptoms. As the neurologist seeks an etiology for the stroke, he asks, "Did you use cocaine today?"

She denies the use of cocaine or any other illicit drugs.

The neurologist then asks, "Would you like your mother to step out of the room for a few minutes?"

Ms. Hawthorne responds, "She can leave, but I still didn't take any cocaine!" She later complains to her mother that she felt insulted by the neurologist's questions.

2   What other approaches could have been used to discuss the issue of illicit drug use with the patient?

Illicit drug use, particularly cocaine and amphetamines, is an important cause of stroke in young people, and it was therefore appropriate to question Ms. Hawthorne about this issue. Given the fear of disclosure by those who might be using/abusing drugs and the possibility of offending those who are free of drugs, it is critical that the question(s) around drug use be properly framed. For example, one might begin by saying:

> The CT scan suggested that you have had a stroke. There are a number of unusual things that may cause a stroke in a young person, so I have to ask you some questions ... "

Further, if there was concern that the mother's presence was preventing the patient from being candid about illicit drug use, then waiting for an opportunity when the mother was out of room to re-address the issue might have been a better approach than asking the mother to "step out."

Ms. Hawthorne is initially treated with aspirin and routine supportive stroke care. A toxicology screen confirmed the absence of any illicit substances, and her pregnancy test was negative. A transesophageal ECG reveals a patent foramen ovale (PFO), but all other tests are normal. After being informed by the resident that she has a "hole" in her heart, Ms. Hawthorne becomes very distressed and tearful and begins to ask several questions. The resident then indicates that the team will discuss the situation with her mother and get back to her. After discussions with her mother, it is decided that a catheter-related, nonsurgical technique will be used to close the PFO.

---

3   What is the basis for the team's paternalistic approach to this patient's treatment, excluding her from the decision-making process?

Legally, patients are assumed to be competent to make medical decisions once they are 18 years and older. However, as adolescent children transition into young adulthood, individual life experiences are different and rates of maturation are not uniform. As a result, the capacity to make medical decisions will vary from one 18-year-old to another and may still be less than complete at this age. This, in turn, may result in the tendency to defer to the parents of legally competent young people. The goal, however, is to respect the autonomy of the young person by beginning the process with him/her and having the parents as a resource that the patient uses to make his or her decision.

A greater challenge is the patient who is younger than 18, particularly in the setting of advanced cancer or end-stage neuromuscular disease and end-of-life decision making. The Committee on Bioethics of the American Academy of Pediatrics has stated, "Decision-making involving the healthcare of older children and adolescents should include to the greatest extent feasible, the assent of that patient." With careful attention to each patient's developmental capacity, rationality, and autonomy, the committee proposed that this could be accomplished by:

- Helping the patient achieve a developmentally appropriate awareness of the nature of his or her condition.
- Telling the patient what he or she can expect with tests and treatments.
- Making a clinical assessment of the patient's understanding of the situation and factors influencing how he or she is responding (including whether there is inappropriate pressure to accept testing or therapy).
- Soliciting an expression of the patient's willingness to accept the proposed care. (The patient's views should only be solicited if they will be seriously considered). Without undermining parental authority or disenfranchising the parents, the goal is that "as children develop, they should gradually become the primary guardians of personal health and the primary partners in medical decision-making, assuming responsibility from their parents."

The Age of Majority

In the past three decades, laws related to medical treatment for minors have changed slowly. In 1971, the age of *"majority"* was changed from 21 to 18; however, in most states, patients under 18 still have no legal rights to participate in medical decision making unless deemed to be "emancipated minors" by virtue of being self-supporting and not living at home, married, in the military, or have petitioned the court to be considered "emancipated." In a few states with "mature minors rules," adolescents over the age of 15 may be treated, without parental involvement, when seeking treatment for contraception, pregnancy, or sexually transmitted diseases.

4   In what way does this case illustrate how a physician's belief or assumption could lead to health-related disparities?

The inappropriate assumptions of the staff ultimately prevented Ms. Hawthorne from receiving stroke-limiting thrombolytic therapy. Multiply these treatment-delaying assumptions many times over in other physicians and nurses with similar beliefs and one could have a health-related disparity in which a potentially significant number of young women do not receive state-of-the art stroke therapy.

Follow-up

During the next few years, the patient recovers substantially from her stroke, graduates from college, and develops a support group for young stroke survivors. She learns that she could have been treated with thrombolytics, had alternative treatment options for her PFO, and regrets not having been able to make her own choices. She now lectures to medical students and other trainees about her misadventures as a patient.

References: Case 21

Committee on Bioethics, American Academy of Pediatrics. Informed consent, parental permission, and assent in pediatric practice. *Pediatrics* 1995;195:314–7.

Goudsmit E. The psychologisation of illness. In : Brostoff J., Challacombe S.J., eds. Food Allergy and Intolerance, 2nd Ed. WB Saunders, Philadelphia, 2002.

Hinds P.S., Drew D., Oakes L.L., et al. End-of-life care preferences of pediatric patients with cancer. *J Clin Oncol* 2005;23(36):9146–54.

Messe S.R., Silverman I.E., Kizer J.R., et al. Practice parameter: recurrent stroke with patent foramen ovale and atrial septal aneurysm: report of the quality standards subcommittee of the American Academy of Neurology. *Neurology* 2004;62:1042–50

Stone J., Carson A., Sharpe M. Functional symptoms and signs in neurology: assessment and diagnosis. *J Neurol Neurosurg Psychiatry* 2005;76:2–12 (suppl 1).

Tobiano P.S., Wang H.E., McCausland J.B., Hammer M.D. A case of conversion disorder presenting as a severe acute stroke. *J Emerg Med* 2006;30:283–6.

Tolat R.D., O' Dell M.W., Golamco-Estrella S.P., Avella H. Cocaine-associated stroke: three cases and rehabilitation considerations. *Brain Inj* 2000;14: 383–91.

Turkoski B.B. When a child's treatment decisions conflict with the parents'. *Home Healthcare Nurse* 2005;23:123–6.

Westover A.N., McBride S., Haley R.W. Stroke in young adults who abuse amphetamines or cocaine: a population-based study of hospitalized patients. *Arch Gen Psychiatry* 2007;64:495–502.

Weir R.F., Peters C. Affirming the decisions adolescents make about life and death. The Hastings Center Report, Vol. 27, 1997.

Zawistowski C.A., Frader J.E. Ethical problems in pediatric critical care: consent. *Crit Care Med* 2003;31(5):S407–10 (suppl).

CASE 22

Alika Nkuutu

A 24-year-old African woman with sickle cell disease

J. Eric Russell, MD

University of Pennsylvania School of Medicine, Philadelphia, PA, USA

Educational Objectives

- Explain the importance of obtaining an interpreter to facilitate effective communication and thus good care.
- Associate previous health-related experiences of individuals from other societies as a possible barrier to their care in America.
- Explain the potential negative consequences of (racial) stereotyping on patient care.
- Discuss how unappreciated cultural beliefs or practices can result in misunderstandings that interfere with patient–physician dialogue.

TACCT Domains: 3, 4, 5

Case Summary, Questions and Answers

Alika Nkuutu is a 24-year-old woman with sickle cell disease who recently arrived from West Africa. She is living in Philadelphia and studying economics at a university in the city. While visiting a cousin in a local suburb, she developed diffuse muscle and joint pains. Despite bed rest and oral hydration, Ms. Nkuutu's discomfort worsened, prompting her to seek treatment at a local hospital Emergency Department (ED) the next evening. She was admitted to the hospital and her pain

---

Achieving Cultural Competency: A case-based approach to training health professionals,
1st edition. Edited by L Hark, H DeLisser. © 2009 Blackwell Publishing,
ISBN: 9781405180726.

> *responded marginally to two intravenous doses of morphine. Ms. Nkuutu was discharged the next morning with a prescription for oxycodone with acetaminophen that she did not fill. Ms. Nkuutu returned to Philadelphia on the weekend and, when her pain persisted, she presented to the ED of the university hospital later that evening in severe painful crisis.*

1 What factors may have caused Ms. Nkuutu to avoid filling the prescription?

A number of factors, including incomplete or erroneous physician instructions, forgetfulness, and/or lack of money or insurance coverage for prescriptions, co-pays, or deductibles, might have contributed to the patient's failure to fill her prescription. It is also important to recognize that health care is organized and delivered differently in the U.S. than many other parts of the world. As a result, experience of illness and its subsequent treatment in the U.S. may be particularly confusing to immigrants from third-world countries. For example, medications in West Africa are commonly obtained in an outdoor market. Thus, Ms. Nkuutu may not have fully understood the purpose or use of a prescription or the practice of obtaining medications from a pharmacy.

2 What initial issues are raised by this patient encounter?

The immediate issues relate to language; specifically, whether a complete evaluation will require the presence of a skilled interpreter. The literature clearly demonstrates that, for patients with limited proficiency in English, the use of a trained interpreter (either on-site or via telephone) results in better heath care experiences, outcomes, and use of services. It is important to remember that patients who speak conversational English may not necessarily understand medical terms or common colloquialisms well enough to provide accurate information or to participate in medical decision making. Additional issues that may be relevant to this encounter, and which might affect treatment plans, include the patient's insurance status, her understanding of American medical culture, and her immigration status (legal/documented vs. illegal/undocumented).

> *Ms. Nkuutu is administered a single intravenous dose of morphine in the ED that provides substantial relief, and is subsequently admitted to an inpatient bed several hours later. During morning rounds, the medical resident states his suspicion that Ms. Nkuutu is exaggerating her pain to obtain narcotics. The resident cites his previous experience with a clinic patient with sickle cell disease who abused hydromorphone hydrochloride, and notes that Ms. Nkuutu is unkempt and half-asleep, and had visited two different EDs in the preceding 24-hour period. A decision is made to start a low dose of morphine and titrate to a higher dose, depending on her response. This plan is questioned when a plasma drug screen indicates the presence of oxycodone. The patient vehemently denies taking any narcotics, which only raises suspicion of drug-seeking behavior and induces the resident to maintain a low dose of morphine that does not effectively treat Ms. Nkuutu's pain. The discrepant results are explained later when Ms. Nkuutu's cousin states that he provided her with two tablets (left over from his recent arthroscopic procedure) without telling her that they contained oxycodone. As this explanation seemed plausible, the patient's morphine dose was increased with an immediate improvement in her pain.*

3   What factors may have contributed to the resident's suspicion of drug-seeking behavior?

The management of vaso-occlusive (acute) pain is a common, yet challenging aspect of sickle cell care. Narcotic dependence (drug-seeking behavior) is observed to occur and remains an important concern for many providers. The suspicion of drug-seeking behavior may affect pain management plans, resulting in premature discharge from the hospital or inadequate postdischarge analgesia. Residents and physicians with limited experience diagnosing painful crisis and acute chest syndromes often look for symptoms or signs that they believe are significant and which match the complaints of pain. Sickle cell pain is not seen in the way a fracture might appear. This, plus stereotyping, often makes the experience of hospitalized sickle cell patients challenging. Therefore, pain treatment is an area where significant disparities exist and formal training can be helpful.

Effective pain management for illnesses, other than sickle cell disease, appears to be subject to racial bias as well. Compared with other groups, racial and ethnic minorities have been noted to receive inadequate pain management in the setting of cancer therapy and while receiving emergency care. The reasons for these disparities are not clear, but may possibly reflect poor doctor–patient interaction or communication.

The matter of stereotyping is significant for patients with sickle cell disease in the United States, more than 90% of whom are African American. In addition to drug-dependency issues discussed above, the burden of chronic disease can interfere with education and/or employment, leading to racial stereotyping of sickle cell patients as drug-seeking, undereducated, unemployed individuals. As the ability to recognize patterns in the patient history and/or examination is central to efficient medical decision making, the fact that the resident used his past experiences to facilitate his current management was not necessarily inappropriate. However, care must be taken to avoid negative stereotyping that could adversely affect patient care. The individuality of each patient should never be sacrificed for the purpose of facilitating efficient diagnosis or therapy.

> *Ms. Nkuutu was cooperative with the medical student and resident at the time of her admission, permitting both to interview and examine her on a daily basis. On the third hospital day, though, Ms. Nkuutu remains fully cooperative with the medical student, but refuses to speak with, or be examined by, the resident. The resident and medical student conclude that the patient's attitude reflects lingering anger surrounding the dosing of the morphine and agree that the medical student should now act as the primary caregiver.*

4 Are there other factors (beside lingering anger) that may have led to the patient's refusal to interact with the medical resident?

Physical actions that have little meaning in Western culture, such as making eye contact, sitting with crossed legs, or extending your left hand in greeting, may have subtle, yet important meanings to individuals raised in other cultures. These nonverbal cues may be highly offensive, intrusive, and/or insensitive in the context of the patient's culture. In the current scenario, the resident extended his left hand in greeting, an act that the patient interpreted to be both offensive and disrespectful. Although the lack of eye contact, or refusal to shake hands, may in fact signify evasiveness or hostility, it is important to recognize that these nonverbal cues may arise from cultural imperatives.

5 Do you agree with the resident's response?

Physicians, particularly those who are training or in the early years of their careers, often feel unprepared to provide cross-cultural care. Although ignorance of cultural issues may reflect deficiencies in medical school curriculum and/or graduate medical training, a physician can defuse many cultural misunderstandings by simply maintaining open and honest communication with patients. In the current case, the resident might have addressed the patient's (assumed) anger by saying, *"I get a sense that you are uncomfortable with me. Can you tell me why?"* Enlisting the services of a trained interpreter, especially someone who is familiar with the patient's cultural background, would probably have been helpful in this case as well.

References: Case 22

Buchanan G.R., DeBaun M.R., Quinn C.T., Steinberg M.H. Sickle cell disease. *Hematology Am Soc Hematol Educ Program* 2004;35–47.

Chen A. Doctoring across the language divide. *Health Aff* 2006;25:808–13.

Djimde A., Plowe C.V., Diop S., Dicko A., Wellems T.E., Doumbo O. Use of antimalarial drugs in Mali: policy versus reality. *Am J Trop Med Hyg* 1998; 59:376–9.

DuPlessis H.M., Cora-Bramble D. American Academy of Pediatrics Committee on Community Health Services. Providing care for immigrant, homeless, and migrant children. *Pediatrics* 2005;115:1095–100.

Elander J., Lusher J., Bevan D., Telfer P. Pain management and symptoms of substance dependence among patients with sickle cell disease. *Soc Sci Med* 2003;57:1683–96.

Elander J., Lusher J., Bevan D., Telfer P., Burton B. Understanding the causes of problematic pain management in sickle cell disease: evidence that pseudoaddiction plays a more important role than genuine analgesic dependence. *J Pain Symptom Manage* 2004;27:156–69.

Flores G. The impact of medical interpreter services on the quality of healthcare: a systematic review. *Med Care Res Rev* 2005;62:255–99.

Grundy R., Howard R., Evans J. Practical management of pain in sickling disorders. *Arch Dis Child* 1993;69(2):256–9.

Hsieh E. Understanding medical interpreters: reconceptualizing bilingual health communication. *Health Commun* 2006;20:177–86.

Okpalak I.E. New therapies for sickle cell disease. *Hematol Oncol Clin North Am* 2005;19:975–87.

Patterson A.E., Winch P.J., Gilroy K.E., Doumbia S. Local terminology for medicines to treat fever in Bougouni District, Mali: implications for the introduction and evaluation of malaria treatment policies. *Trop Med Int Health* 2006;11:1613–24.

Romero C.M. Using medical interpreters. *Am Fam Physician* 2004;69:2720–2.

Stauffer W.M., Kamat D., Walker P.F. Screening of international immigrants, refugees, and adoptees. *Prim Care* 2002;29:879–905.

Stuart M.J., Nagel R.L. Sickle-cell disease. *Lancet* 2004;364:1343–60.

Switzer J.A., Hess D.C., Nichols F.T., Adams R.J. Pathophysiology and treatment of stroke in sickle-cell disease: present and future. *Lancet Neurol* 2006;5:501–12.

Tavrow P., Shabahang J., Makama S. Vendor-to-vendor education to improve malaria treatment by private drug outlets in Bungoma District, Kenya. *Malar J* 2003;2:10.

Todd K.H., Green C., Bonham V.L., Haywood C., Ivy E. Sickle cell disease related pain: crisis and conflict. *J Pain* 2006;7:453–8.

Weissman J.S., Betancourt J., Campbell E.G., et al. Resident physicians' preparedness to provide cross-cultural care. *JAMA* 2005;294:1058–67.

CASE 23

Miguel Cortez

A 9-year-old Mexican boy with asthma

Noel B. Rosales, MD
Children's Hospital of Philadelphia, Philadelphia, PA, USA

Educational Objectives

- Describe how to effectively use a trained medical interpreter.
- Express some of the challenges that arise in using a medical interpreter.
- Explain how sociocultural factors may influence the health care decisions of patients.

TACCT Domains: 4, 5, 6

Case Summary, Questions and Answers

Miguel Cortez is a 9-year-old Mexican immigrant with asthma who comes with his mother for the first time to the outpatient general pediatric clinic to follow-up on his recent hospitalization for an asthma exacerbation, about 1 month ago. Whereas Miguel is fluent in Spanish and English and reads English, his mother, Adela Cortez, does not speak English. The pediatrician, Dr. Eisen, enters the room and greets Mrs. Cortez, asking how Miguel is feeling. The mother looks at Miguel and asks him in Spanish, "What is the doctor saying?" Without answering his mother, Miguel tells Dr. Eisen, "I am fine," without elaborating further. Dr. Eisen again turns to Miguel's mother and asks, "Is he really fine?" With embarrassment she responds, "No English."

Achieving Cultural Competency: A case-based approach to training health professionals, 1st edition. Edited by L Hark, H DeLisser. © 2009 Blackwell Publishing, ISBN: 9781405180726.

1   What issues arise when conducting a medical evaluation of a 9-year-old child without an interpreter if his mother does not speak English?

Relying on this 9-year-old to speak for himself instead of obtaining an interpreter is certainly very problematic for a number of reasons. Obviously, children at this age, even very intelligent ones, lack the sophistication and communication skills to adequately respond to medical-related questions and/or may have trouble recalling important details, such as the onset, duration, and frequency of his/her own symptoms. Further, 9-year-old children may also lack awareness and insight, which may prevent them from providing accurate information about their own condition. For example, it is not uncommon to see a 9-year-old child with severe asthma and little air movement who will tell you that nothing is wrong. There is, however, a more fundamental concern. Allowing the child to speak for himself, while excluding the mother, has the potential of creating a sense of inadequacy in the mother and marginalizing her as a parent as well as harms the child by parentifying him (or setting adult expectations inappropriate for a child). This change in the power dynamic ultimately may undermine the parent–child relationship and/or contribute to future adherence problems.

2   Why is it important to use a trained medical interpreter when working with patients who do not speak English?

Medical interpretation may be provided by ad hoc interpreters (family members, friends or available, untrained medical or nonmedical staff), trained/professional interpreters, or telephone interpreter services. There is ample evidence that, for patients with limited English proficiency (LEP), the use of trained interpreters (either on-site or via telephone) results in better heath care experiences, outcomes, and the use of services. A skilled, trained interpreter ideally transmits information in a seamless way between the clinician and the patient as accurately as possible with minimal distortion. If done well, these trained interpreters can further help to simplify medical information in a way that ensures the patient understands what the clinician is trying to say, teach, or advise. Their previous experiences with medical terminology can further help to facilitate the conversation. Although there are admittedly unavoidable situations, given the above, the use of ad hoc interpreters is not encouraged.

Having said all of this, some of the potential limitations should be noted. First, it is important to acknowledge the challenges faced by a trained interpreter in faithfully acting as a neutral, two-way conduit of information, behavior which, although expected, some would argue is not always desirable. Second, the language barrier and the presence of an interpreter inevitably tends to stifle some of the purely social and spontaneous interactions, "small talk," that could and does occur between patient and physician who communicate directly to each other in the same language. For groups where this kind of interaction is important, its absence may diminish some of their satisfaction with the physician encounter. Aranguri and colleagues also suggest that the lack of social discourse limits the physician's ability to diagnose any psychosocial disorders or compliance/adherence issues related to the social situation of LEP patients. Appendix 1 describes how to effectively position an interpreter.

> *Upon learning that Mrs. Cortez does not speak English, Dr. Eisen arranged for a hospital provided interpreter to join the interview. Through the interpreter, Mrs. Cortez reported that, when Miguel was discharged from the hospital, he had been prescribed fluticasone and albuterol. Upon discharge, because she did not speak English and an interpreter was not available, she was given written instructions in Spanish. These instructions explained that Miguel should continue the medicine every day in order to suppress the inflammation and prevent future asthma exacerbations. She admitted that as Miguel was feeling better, she stopped giving these medications over the last 2 weeks.*

3 Why might Mrs. Cortez have stopped giving Miguel his asthma medications?

One potential issue is how the discharge instructions were explained to the patient and parent. When providing written instructions to patients and/or families, their literacy level and ability to read should not necessarily be assumed as it is not valid to assume that literacy exists in every patient. This is particularly important for immigrant populations, where the educational opportunities in their native country may have been limited. In this case, Miguel's mother received discharge summary instructions that were written in Spanish, assuming that she was literate in Spanish. In fact, Mrs. Cortez is unable to read (Spanish) and, therefore, did not understand the inflammatory nature of asthma and the need to continue the steroids (i.e. fluticasone) to maintain suppression of the airway inflammation. Certainly in this situation, it would have been important to have an interpreter to provide her with verbal instructions.

Other issues beyond the lack of proper instructions that have to be considered include the influence of native beliefs about the nature, cause, and treatment of asthma, or lung diseases in general, and a fear of her child being harmed by or becoming "addicted" to the medications. The possible importance of these additional factors to immigrant health in the U.S. is highlighted by the study of Bearison and colleagues, who surveyed mothers from a Dominican American community regarding their beliefs about asthma and asthma treatment. It was noted that most mothers in this group of Hispanic women (72%) reported that they did not use prescribed medicines for the prevention of asthma, instead substituting home remedies derived from their folk beliefs about health and illness. Further, nearly two-thirds thought their children did not have asthma in the absence of an acute exacerbation, and 88% believed that medications were overprescribed.

> *Through the interpreter, the physician asks mom if Miguel is wheezing ("Jadeo") at night. The clinician notices that mom seems puzzled by the word Jadeo. She says to the interpreter in Spanish, "What do you mean?" Despite further effort on the part of the interpreter to clarify the question, she still does not understand what is being asked.*

4   Why might Mrs. Cortez have trouble understanding the concept of wheezing when asked by the interpreter?

Mrs. Cortez is Hispanic, specifically Mexican. The term "Hispanic" refers to ethnicity and not race and is defined by the federal government as including a person of Mexican, Puerto Rican, Cuban, South or Central American, or other Spanish culture or origin. According to the U.S. Census Bureau, as of census 2000, there were 37.4 million Hispanics in the U.S., which constituted 13.3% of the population. Current data suggest that Puerto Ricans have higher prevalence and

Table 23.1 An informal sampling of Spanish words used to describe wheezing

Spanish word	May be used in	Comments/translation
Pito, peruvia	Mexico	"Whistling sound"
Ronquer		"Snoring"
Jadeo	Cuba	"Panting"
Resuello, Silbido	Puerto Rico	
Sibilancia	Dominican Republic	
Hervor de pecho	Central American	"Boiling in the chest"

Source: Noel Rosales, MD, The Children's Hospital of Philadelphia, 2009. Used with Permission.

mortality rates of asthma than other ethnic groups or other Hispanic subgroups, whereas Mexican Americans appear to have a lower risk of asthma compared with other groups.

As in all languages, there are different dialects and word usages in Spanish that can create challenges when trying to understand the patient's symptoms, even when an interpreter is being employed. For example, the English word "wheezing" does not directly translate into one Spanish word and so it is expressed differently depending on the patient's particular Spanish. (Table 23.1) Similarly, instructing the patient to take "two puffs" from their inhaler may not be easily interpreted as shown in Table 23.2. Therefore, it is usually helpful to ask the patient what words they use to describe a particular symptom.

> *Miguel is started again on fluticasone and albuterol, and an asthma care plan is formulated. Using a trained medical interpreter, the care plan is explained in both Spanish and English so both the mother and Miguel can follow it. Mrs. Cortez is able to demonstrate her understanding of the care plan by using a "teach back" approach, where her understanding of the treatment is confirmed by having her repeat back what was instructed. If there appears to be misunderstanding or confusion, the instructions or information are again repeated, presumably in a way that better facilitates their understanding, and the patient/family once again is asked to describe what they have heard. The process is repeated until understanding has been achieved.*

> However, over the next several months, despite adherence to the treatment plan, Miguel's asthma becomes difficult to control. Because of this, Dr. Eisen wants to enroll Miguel and his family in an asthma care program that includes home visits to assess for environmental triggers for asthma. It is explained (through an interpreter) that the program is free of charge and could greatly benefit Miguel, but Mrs. Cortez becomes very defensive and adamantly refuses to participate in the program. Despite vigorous encouragement, Dr. Eisen is unable to convince Mrs. Cortez to enroll in this initiative and is very puzzled by her refusal.

5   Why might Mrs. Cortez refuse to participate in this program?

There may be undocumented immigrants at home, and so Mrs. Cortez may be reluctant to enroll in this program because of a fear that strangers entering the house might discover these individuals and report them to the authorities. This concern about being reported may lead undocumented immigrants to delay seeking medical treatment or result in incomplete disclosure of relevant medical or personal information. This is an example of a psychosocial issue that, along with biological and environmental factors, might increase the morbidity of asthma in Hispanics.

Table 23.2 For "two puffs" of an inhaled medication from a metered dose inhaler

Spanish phrase	English translation
Dos inhalaciones	Two inhalations
Dos pulsaciones	Two pulsations
Dos puffs	Two puffs
Dos Sprays	Two sprays
Dos Soplos	Two blows
Usar in bomba dos veces	Use the pump two times
Dos apretatas de inhalador	Two squeezes of the inhaler
Dos empujadas de inhalador	Two pushes of the inhaler
Inhalar dos disparos	Inhale two blasts or firings

Source: Noel Rosales, MD, The Children's Hospital of Philadelphia, 2009. Used with Permission.

References: Case 23

Aranguri C., Davidson B., Ramirez R. Patterns of communication through interpreters: a detailed sociolinguistic analysis. *J Gen Intern Med* 2006;21:623–9.

Bearison D.J., Minian N., Granowetter L. Medical management of asthma and folk medicine in a Hispanic community. *J Pediatr Psychol* 2002;27(4):385–92.

Chen A. Doctoring across the language divide. *Health Aff* 2006;25:808–13.

Cohen R.T., Celedon J.C. Asthma in Hispanics in the United States. *Clin Chest Med* 2006;27:401–12.

Dysart-Gale D. Communication, models, professionalism, and the work of medical interpreters. *Health Commun* 2005;17:91–103.

Earley L, Cushway D. The parentified child. *Clin Child Psychol Psychiatry* 2002;7(2):163–78.

Flores G. The impact of medical interpreter services on the quality of healthcare: a systematic review. *Med Care Res Rev* 2005;62:255–99.

Horne R. Compliance, adherence, and concordance: implications for asthma treatment. *Chest* 2006;130(1:65S–72S (suppl).

Hsieh E. Conflicts in how interpreters manage their roles in provider-patient interactions. *Soc Sci Med* 2006;62:721–30.

Hsieh E. Understanding medical interpreters: reconceptualizing bilingual health communication. *Health Commun* 2006;20:177–86.

Romero C.M. Using medical interpreters. *Am Fam Physician* 2004;69:2720–2.

Szelfer S.J. Advances in pediatric asthma. *J Allergy Clin Immunol* 2007;121(3):614–9.

Naomi Fulton

A 49-year-old African American woman with metabolic syndrome

Gail Marion, PA-C, PhD,[1] *and Lisa Hark, PhD, RD*[2]

[1] Wake Forest University School of Medicine, Winston-Salem, PA, USA
[2] Jefferson Medical College, Philadelphia, PA, USA

Educational Objectives

- Acknowledge that many people in the African American community view being overweight/obese as desirable from both an aesthetic and health perspective.
- Share with patients that over 50% of African American women are obese and that metabolic syndrome and diabetes are increasing rapidly in minority populations.
- Learn to use the 5 A's model to assess patient's readiness to change and their conviction and confidence to modify lifestyles and adhere to treatment recommendations.

TACCT Domains: 1, 2, 4

Case Summary, Questions and Answers

Ms. Naomi Fulton is a 49-year-old African American woman who comes to see her family doctor, Dr. Clark, for an annual physical. She works as a teacher's aid in a middle school and is a music director for her local church. Ms. Fulton is 5'4" and weighs 190 lbs (BMI = 33). Her waist

Achieving Cultural Competency: A case-based approach to training health professionals, 1st edition. Edited by L Hark, H DeLisser. © 2009 Blackwell Publishing, ISBN: 9781405180726.

*circumference is 40 inches. Her blood pressure on three separate oc-
casions averages 130/90 mm Hg. Her average fasting blood sugar is
118 mg/dL. Dr. Clark diagnoses her with metabolic syndrome and explains that diet and exercise are the most effective treatments to reduce her chances of developing diabetes and heart disease. She also
explains to Ms. Fulton that her health will improve significantly if she
loses weight by eating less and exercising more. Dr. Clark tells Ms. Fulton
that an ideal weight for her is 125 lbs. Ms. Fulton agrees to try and is
given a follow-up appointment in 3 months.*

1 What information was missing from this encounter?

Even though studies show that weight reduction and increasing
physical activity are effective treatments for many of the abnormalities associated with metabolic syndrome, instructing a patient to eat
less and exercise more has not been shown to be effective in getting
patients to change their lifestyle behaviors. Although this message
is simple, helping patients to change their diet and lifestyle requires
clinicians to use effective counseling skills to actually achieve modi-
fiable goals. In order to effectively improve a patient's diet, the clinician needs to spend a few minutes obtaining a diet history. This
includes asking the patient either what they usually eat and drink
during a typical day or asking them to recall everything they ate
and drank the day before the visit. When evaluating this information, look for food groups that are missing or excessive. For example,
many patients do not eat the recommended five servings of vegetables, four servings of fruits, or three servings of low-fat dairy foods
every day. They may also be eating too much saturated fat and protein, or including an excess amount of foods and beverages high in
sugar or artificial sweeteners.

In addition, since increasing physical activity, especially walking,
can reduce waist circumference and the risk of diabetes, heart disease, hypertension, and several types of cancer, it is critical to also
assess a patient's activity level and sedentary behaviors. "How often do they exercise?" including walking each day, and "how many
hours each day do they spend watching television?" Current recommendations from the *U.S. Dietary Guidelines for Adult Americans* advise
at least 30 minutes of physical activity per day to reduce the risk of
chronic diseases; at least 60 minutes per day to prevent weight gain;

and 60 to 90 minutes per day to lose weight. It is recommended that screen time (television, video and computer games) be limited to less than 2 hours per day.

It is important to determine the patient's and her family's attitudes about her current weight and activity level; how comfortable is she with her current body weight, and are there any other issues regarding her weight that she wants to share? For example, has she ever tried to lose weight or start an exercise program and what has been her experience if she has made previous efforts? This will help to identify barriers to changing her diet and increasing her exercise level.

2   Is this goal weight realistic for Ms. Fulton? Why or why not?

Discussing weight with patients is important, but Dr. Clark's approach has not been helpful or effective. In a recent study of 12,000 overweight and obese patients, 58% said that they never discussed weight with their primary care physician (PCP). When clinicians do give weight-loss counseling, it *triples* the odds that patients will attempt to lose weight. However, asking Ms. Fulton or any other patient to lose 65 lbs, or 30% of her body weight, is not only an unrealistic weight goal, but not necessary to modify risk factors for metabolic syndrome. Studies show that patients may only need to lose 5% to 10% of their body weight (10 to 20 lbs for Mrs. Fulton) to improve their blood pressure, blood sugar, and blood cholesterol levels and reduce their waist circumference.

> *Ms. Fulton returns to the office 3 months later for an evaluation. She has not lost any weight. Her blood pressure is 138/90 mm Hg and her blood sugar is 120 mg/dL. Dr. Clark asks her if she would like a referral for a nutritionist to help with weight loss and reminds her that an ideal weight for her would be 125 lbs and, therefore, she needs to lose 65 lbs.*

3   How could this second encounter have been improved?

Dr. Clark simply repeats what did not work at the first visit. Further, she fails to explore why Ms. Fulton has been unsuccessful at losing weight. In order to improve this encounter, she should listen respectfully to Ms. Fulton's statements of resistance (or commitment) to change and reflect these back to her. Eliciting the pros and cons of behavior change from Mrs. Fulton is part of a technique called motivational interviewing, which has been shown to be an effective strategy at helping people change behavior. Collaborate and reach agreement on goals that match this patient's stage of change. Begin by assessing Mrs. Fulton's conviction and confidence with respect to improving her diet and exercise habits. Explore these questions:

- What is her understanding of metabolic syndrome?
- Does she understand the significance of her metabolic syndrome diagnosis?
- Does she identify that this is a health problem for her?
- Does she understand the relationship between her diet, physical activity, and her diagnosis and is she willing to make changes?
- How confident is Ms. Fulton that she can make the necessary changes to her lifestyle?
- How do her family, current partner, and culture view ideal body types?

It is best to avoid attempting to persuade patients who have a low level of conviction to change their behavior because this will likely only upset or alienate patients. Avoid trying to direct or pre-scribe action plans when patients state that they are unwilling to change or they lack confidence. The best approach is to document the patient's current stage of change and readdress the topic at a future visit, particularly when there may be a teachable moment (e.g. increased knee pain secondary to excess weight or a new diagnosis of diabetes in a patient who has metabolic syndrome). By evaluating Ms. Fulton's perspective on her health and enabling her to identify what she is most likely to do first as an intervention, the physician enables her to take concrete actions that are realistic, feasible, and crafted and framed by the patient rather than the physician.

Ms. Fulton returns to the office 3 months later and again has not lost any weight. Her blood pressure is slightly worse at 135/90 mm Hg and her fasting blood sugar is 118 mg/dL. She says that she visited the nutritionist and found it helpful, but she did not know how successful she was going to be because her husband likes her the way she is. Dr. Clark realizes that this is a barrier to losing weight and initiates a discussion with Ms. Fulton. She says she is embarrassed to admit that he likes her body to be full-figured, and does not know how to change her husband's feelings about her figure.

4   How can this issue be addressed with Ms. Fulton?

Acknowledging Ms. Fulton's discomfort about her husband's preferences in a respectful manner will help to make her feel more comfortable with modest weight loss. What kind of conversations have
she and her husband had about this issue and how can Dr. Clark
begin to understand the dynamics of this couple about her health
and her weight? Dr. Clark could begin the conversation by saying:

> *"I appreciate the fact that you are sharing this very private informa-
> tion with me, and I know it is not easy to admit that he prefers you
> stay the way you are. Have you discussed with your husband your re-
> cent metabolic syndrome diagnosis and desire to improve your health?
> Would you be willing to bring Mr. Fulton with you for your next
> scheduled appointment?"*

From a gender perspective, the physician can also reinforce that he
or she is not defining health as being skinny, but only emphasizing
that excess weight around the abdomen contributes to metabolic
syndrome, cardiovascular disease, diabetes, and certain types of
cancer.

5   If Ms. Fulton brings her husband to the office at the next visit, what would be the most appropriate way to discuss his attitudes about her weight?

Begin by exploring Mr. Fulton's perspectives on his wife's body
weight, both from an aesthetic as well as a health perspective. Recognize that he too may be overweight and sedentary. It is important
to acknowledge that changing a diet from usual, familiar, high-fat
comfort foods to those less familiar or perceived as "healthy" may
be difficult at first. Ask how much weight his wife could lose before
he would find her less attractive. Ask him to consider his aesthetic
perspectives and balance these with long-term health consequences
of remaining obese. Based on his comments, educate him about
the health risks associated with being overweight and obese and
her recent diagnosis of metabolic syndrome. Stress that metabolic
syndrome represents an opportunity to intervene early as a way to
prevent and reduce the risk of developing diabetes, cardiovascular
disease, and certain cancers.

The same steps used to understand the patient's confidence and
conviction can be used for the encounter with her spouse. Listen
respectfully to Mr. Fulton's statements of resistance (or commitment) to change and reflect these back to him. Collaborate and reach

agreement on goals that match this couple's stage of change, conviction, and confidence. Once again, using motivational interviewing to have them identify what is realistic and likely to change regarding diet and exercise is a useful technique to employ. Asking them to summarize what changes they think they can make, noting these in the plan and sharing a copy of the note with the patient and her husband will facilitate continuity for the next visit and reinforce the efforts they are willing to make.

Motivational Interviewing

Motivational interviewing, described by its creators as "a way of being with people," is a communication strategy that has been shown to be effective in helping patients modify addictive behaviors and is increasingly being applied in a variety of clinical settings. The goal of motivational interviewing is to understand what the motivational state of the client is at the time and to act appropriately. For example, in the precontemplation stage, a person needs information and feedback to better understand the problem and to begin to imagine that change is possible. Giving advice at this point is not helpful.

Motivational interviewing is characterized by eliciting motivation from the client, not trying to impose it from the outside. It has been defined as a directive, client-centered counseling style for eliciting behavior change by helping clients to explore and resolve ambivalence. Resolving ambivalence is a key to motivational interviewing.

When people move into the contemplation stage, when they are thinking about changing vs. not changing, balancing out the pros and cons, they are more susceptible to real change. However, a helping professional who starts pushing behavior change at the client at this stage will meet resistance. It is the client's task, not the counselor's, to identify and resolve his or her ambivalence. What the client needs at this point is help listing pros and cons and a nonjudgmental, encouraging professional who really listens. The client determines whether his/her current behavior is consistent with goals and then makes choices to move him or herself. The traditional advice-giving, confrontation, and authority, so often employed in the medical setting, have been shown to be less effective than motivational interviewing in resolving ambivalence and promoting change. Piling up arguments for the pro change side will leave the client the role of piling up arguments for the con side of change. Rather, the provider is there to assist the client in exploring the pros and cons.

The counseling style is generally a quiet, supportive, and eliciting one. In this setting, effective patient education requires more active listening than talking. Readiness to change is not a client trait but a fluctu-ating product of interpersonal interaction. The therapeutic relation-ship is more like a partnership than one of expert/recipient, and good provider–client rapport is crucial for success. Patient motivation requires establishing a therapeutic relationship from which motivation can grow. Motivational interviewing brief intervention tools are being increas-ingly employed in the primary care setting as part of a patient-centered communication strategy. Patient-centered communication is character-ized by partnership building, empathy, interpersonal sensitivity, and in-formation giving – all highly consistent with the central tenets of moti-vational interviewing. These strategies have been shown to increase pa-tient satisfaction, treatment adherence, and disclosure of psychosocial concerns. To complement motivational interviewing-based interviews, confidence and importance rating scales are often useful. The scales are used during or at the end of the visit, when a provider might ask: "On a scale of 1 to 10, how important do you feel it is to follow the plan we discussed?" (e.g. to take this medicine or to go to this appointment) "And, how confident do you feel that you can do this?" (e.g. remember portion sizes as no larger than the palm of your hand or being able to keep the nutritionist's appointment.).

References: Case 24

Anuura E., Chiem A., Pearson T.A., Berglund L. Metabolic syndrome com-ponents in African-Americans and European-American patients and its relation to coronary artery disease. *Am J Cardiol* 2007;100(5):830–4.

Appel S.J., Moore T.M., Giger J.N. An overview and update on the metabolic syndrome: implications for identifying cardiometabolic risk among African-American women. *J Natl Black Nurses Assoc* 2006;17(2):47–62.

Chen W., Srinivasan S.R., Li S., Xu J., Berenson G.S. Clustering of long-term trends in metabolic syndrome variables from childhood to adult-hood in blacks and whites: the Bogalusa Heart Study. *Am J Epidemiol* 2007;166(5):527–33.

Clark L.T., El-Atat F. Metabolic syndrome in African Americans: implications for preventing coronary heart disease. *Clin Cardiol* 2007;30(4):161–4.

Ekelund U., Brage S., Franks P.W., Hennings S., Emms S., Wareham N.J. Physical activity energy expenditure predicts progression toward the metabolic syndrome independently of aerobic fitness in middle-aged healthy Caucasians: the Medical Research Council Ely Study. *Diabetes Care* 2005;28(5):1195–200.

Giugliano D., Ceriello A., Esposito K. Are there specific treatments for the metabolic syndrome? *Am J Clin Nutr* 2008;87(1):8–11.

Lin S.X., Pi-Sunyer E.X. Prevalence of the metabolic syndrome among US middle-aged and older adults with and without diabetes–a preliminary analysis of the NHANES 1999–2002 data. *Ethn Dis* 2007;17(1):35–9.

Loucks E.B., Rehkopf D.H., Thurston R.C., Kawachi I. Socioeconomic disparities in metabolic syndrome differ by gender: evidence from NHANES III. *Ann Epidemiol* 2007;17(1):19–26.

Miller W.R., Rollnick S. *Motivational Interviewing: Preparing People for Change*, 2nd ed. Guilford Publishing, New York, 2002.

Oh E.G., Hyun S.S., Kim S.H., et al. A randomized controlled trial of therapeutic lifestyle modification in rural women with metabolic syndrome: a pilot study. *Metabolism* 2008;57(2):255–61.

Rankins J., Wortham J., Brown L.L. Modifying soul food for the dietary approaches to stop hypertension diet (DASH) plan: implications for metabolic syndrome (DASH of Soul). *Ethn Dis* 2007;17(3):S4–12 (suppl 4).

Ribisl P.M., Lang W., Jaramillo S.A., et al. Look AHEAD Research Group. Exercise capacity and cardiovascular/metabolic characteristics of overweight and obese individuals with type 2 diabetes: the Look AHEAD clinical trial. *Diabetes Care* 2007;30(10):2679–84.

Serdula M.K., Khan L.K., Dietz W.H. Weight loss counseling revisited. *JAMA* 2003;289(14)1747–50.

Vigneri P., Frasca F., Sciacca L., Frittitta L., Vigneri R. Evidence of the association between increased BMI and the risk of increased cancer incidence in human subjects. Obesity and cancer. *Nutr Metab Cardio Dis* 2006;16:1–7.

Williams R.A., Flack J.M., Gavin J.R., Schneider W.R., Hennekens C.H. Guidelines for management of high-risk African Americans with multiple cardiovascular risk factors: recommendations of an expert consensus panel. *Ethn Dis* 2007;17(2):214–20.

CASE 25

Bobby Napier

A 68-year-old Caucasian Appalachian man with type 2 diabetes

Elizabeth Lee-Rey, MD, MPH,[1] Sonia Crandall, PhD, MS,[2] and Thomas A. Arcury, PhD[2]

[1] Albert Einstein College of Medicine, Bronx, NY, USA
[2] Wake Forest University School of Medicine, Winston-Salem, NC, USA

Educational Objectives

- Identify the impact of socioeconomic factors on access to care.
- Define the religious beliefs that may influence health-seeking behaviors of patients.
- Associate how past experience with the health care system affects the patient's attitudes.
- Illustrate the similarities in the health care experiences of patients from rural communities and inner-city settings.

TACCT Domains: 2, 3, 4, 6

Case Summary, Questions and Answers

Mr. Napier is a 68-year-old Caucasian man with type 2 diabetes who lives in a rural Appalachian county. He and his wife have come to a small primary care center in the neighboring county for a checkup. He is seen by a resident, Dr. John Cox, who is doing a month-long rural medicine rotation. Mrs. Napier tells Dr. Cox that she is concerned that her husband is shuffling his feet when he walks, but Mr. Napier denies

Achieving Cultural Competency: A case-based approach to training health professionals, 1st edition. Edited by L Hark, H DeLisser. © 2009 Blackwell Publishing, ISBN: 9781405180726.

having any problems. Mr. Napier smokes about a pack of cigarettes each day and has smoked or chewed tobacco since his early teens. He does not drink alcohol. At his last visit to the center over a year ago, Mr. Napier complained of burning in his feet, polyuria, and some blurred vision. His random blood glucose 1 year ago was 215 mg/dL (<200 mg/dL) and HbA1c was 11% (normal 4.8% to 6.4%). He was prescribed Metformin, but admits that he only filled the prescription once. Today's 2-hour post-prandial glucose fingerstick result is 290 mg/dL. Dr. Cox then accuses Mr. Napier of neglecting his health, specifically citing his refusal to take his medications, monitor his glucose, quit smoking, or change his diet. Dr. Cox states angrily, "Your diabetes is so out of control! If you keep ignoring what you eat and don't start monitoring your blood sugars regularly, you are going to lose a leg!"

1 How might the attitude that Dr. Cox expressed to Mr. Napier affect his care?

Although Dr. Cox may have been concerned about Mr. Napier's health, his response was inappropriate and unprofessional. Dr. Cox failed to establish a rapport with Mr. Napier and took his denial of anything being wrong as evidence that Mr. Napier was disinterested in his health. Dr. Cox also did not appreciate that this visit was likely initiated by his wife. He instead chose to react to laboratory results, providing unsolicited advice, and resorting to fear. Therefore, Dr. Cox's attitude could irreparably damage his ability to develop a relationship with both Mr. and Mrs. Napier and may cause Mr. Napier to be even more reluctant to seek or receive appropriate medical care.

2 What are some of the factors that need to be considered when prescribing treatment for patients who are poor?

Factors that influence adherence to treatment include a patient's insurance status, access to locally available health care and educational programs, convenient and reliable transportation, and ability to pay for medications either out of pocket or by payment assistance. All of these factors are relevant to Mr. Napier.

If asked, Dr. Cox would have learned that Mr. Napier lives 15 miles away from the nearest pharmacy, and the closest hospital is a small, rural primary care center located in the next county. He was prescribed diabetes medications last year, but these are expensive and Mr. Napier does not have sufficient income or insurance coverage to pay for these medications. His lack of health care insurance arises from the fact that although Mr. Napier is eligible for government sponsored coverage, he has refused this type of assistance, calling it welfare. Mr. Napier's lack of adequate insurance leads to lack of access to resources such as diabetes prevention and educational programs. Together these factors have made it difficult for him to follow through on his diabetes management at home.

The county health department has limited group programs for people with diabetes, but it would require regular travel to the county seat. There is a comprehensive diabetes program in a state university medical center approximately 70 miles from Mr. Napier's home. Mr. Napier's car is old and not dependable for traveling much farther than the county seat. All of his children and their spouses work, and it is difficult for them to take time off to transport Mr. Napier to the university diabetes program.

> *Dr. Cox presents Mr. Napier to Dr. Jennings, the supervising attending physician at the center and says, "Mr. Napier is a noncompliant patient. He was last seen here 1 year ago and doesn't seem at all interested in controlling his diabetes! Frankly, I have other patients who care more about their health who are waiting to be seen, so I don't want to waste anymore time with him."*

3   What would be an appropriate response from the attending to Dr. Cox's statements about Mr. Napier?

This is an opportunity for Dr. Jennings to challenge Dr. Cox's impression of Mr. Napier. This can be done by asking Dr. Cox to elaborate on his conclusions, with the goal of helping him to understand that ethical and professional obligations require him to try to understand the patient's lack of adherence. Effective physician–patient interactions are not, "I say-you do." Dr. Jennings can give feedback on Dr. Cox's communication style by inquiring about what he knows about Mr. Napier's understanding of his diabetes and what he views he can realistically do to control his symptoms. As Dr. Cox has not addressed these questions, Dr. Jennings can help him reframe the encounter to improve the interaction. Part of this process is to accept that Mr. Napier has returned to the health center with the intention of receiving treatment for his medical problems. Unfortunately, whenever the patient's and the health care provider's treatment plans are not aligned, the patient is often labeled as "noncompliant."

These are the kinds of labels that may prevent health care providers from truly understanding their patients.

4   What additional information would have been helpful to Dr. Cox in developing a treatment plan?

A thorough and detailed social and family history obtained in a culturally sensitive, thoughtful, and respectful manner is essential to understanding the particular challenges and obstacles that limit Mr. Napier's care and reduce his ability to adhere to prescribed treatment. To discuss a therapeutic plan with Mr. Napier and his family without understanding the ecological/environmental context of his life will negatively affect communication, cause frustration for everyone involved, delay care, and worsen his health outcomes.

Mr. Napier and his wife have been married for 49 years and have never spent a night apart while married. In addition to raising their six children, the Napier's have worked together throughout their lives, whether in the garden, cutting tobacco, or building their new house. Mr. Napier lives on 500 acres of mountain land that he owns, and his house is on land adjacent to the farm on which he was raised. Four of his six children live on plots of land he has given them; he can see their homes from his front porch. He has walked on and knows all the land in this valley and the surrounding ridges. He knows everyone who lives in the neighborhood. Many of the older residents have been his friends since youth. Many of the younger residents call him Uncle Bobby, whether or not they are actually related.

He has never made more than $10,000 in any year of his life. However, he has worked hard his entire life and supported his family by selling tobacco and vegetables from his garden. Mr. Napier's cash income came from operating a small portable lumber mill (he cut and sold railroad ties), producing tobacco sticks used in the production of burley tobacco, and driving a school bus.

5   How might the social information obtained above be used to promote adherence to his diabetes treatments?

Mr. Napier is a resourceful fellow and has been industrious, given his limited means. Asking him what he would suggest if one of his family members or friends had problems with burning feet, excessive urination, and blurred vision might help him to see his diabetes in a new light. Additionally, sharing your opinion with him about his ability to problem solve, which is now needed regarding his health issues, might be useful. He is not only a dedicated family man with close-knit family members (who may also have diabetes or may help him change his behavior), he is also an important and valued member of the local community. Consequently, enlisting the support of members of his family or his community (while acknowledging his pride in strength and autonomy) may also be beneficial.

> *Dr. Jennings and Dr. Cox return to the exam room to talk to Mr. and Mrs. Napier about his diabetes; however, they have both left the clinic. Dr. Jennings was told by the receptionist that Mr. Napier was upset with the way he was spoken to by Dr. Cox. Three days later, Mr. Napier is brought to the Emergency Department (ED) in the neighboring county after falling from a ladder while picking peaches. Mr. Napier is seen by Dr. Joiner, the family medicine resident on call, who tells Mr. Napier and his son that he has a broken ankle and an elevated blood glucose level of 472 mg/dL. After having his ankle cast, Mr. Napier is admitted to the hospital for management of his diabetes and followed by Dr. Joiner.*

6 What are some of the things that could be done to increase the likelihood that Mr. Napier's diabetes will be controlled in the future?

The management of diabetes requires a multidisciplinary approach, one that includes the patient, the family, health care providers, and resources that will facilitate effective negotiation of the health care delivery system. An assessment of Mr. Napier's understanding of diabetes and its significance to his health and lifestyle is necessary before interventions can be offered and discussed. After reading the patient's chart and conferring with the resident, the attending asked Mr. Napier what his blood sugar readings have been and what his blood sugar goals should be. Mr. Napier admits that he has no idea! Dr. Joiner also needs to assess Mr. Napier's beliefs and understandings about his diabetes and health in general (i.e. illicit Mr. Napier's explanatory model of illness; see appendix) in order to enlist Mr. Napier's critical participation in his care.

It is important to recognize that issues such as smoking cessation, risk for poor healing, and potential complications from an ankle fracture are germane to his care and must be addressed. This should be done in a culturally appropriate manner that recognizes the importance of the sociocultural and economic reality of Mr. Napier's life and experiences, which include raising tobacco as both a source of income and pleasure. Unfortunately, in every instance, the interventions that were offered to him did not take into consideration Mr. Napier, his family, or support systems. In rural Appalachia, poverty and its resultant burden of scarce resources further limit access to care. The connection to land is sacred and the pride of self-sufficiency and reliance on family and church remain the core of Appalachian life. Mr. Napier's story appears to be a reflection of this.

It will be important for Dr. Joiner to identify resources that are available for Mr. Napier and his family. A doctor cannot expect a patient to adhere to treatment if the patient lacks basic health literacy. A recent study (see Smith and Tessaro, 2005) that looked at patient-perceived barriers to preventive health care in diabetes among indigent, rural Appalachian patients found that there was a lack of knowledge about diabetes before and after their diagnosis and a lack of awareness of the risk of diabetes (absent family history). Participants in this study also reported insufficient information about diet, physical activity, and other resources, such as affordable diabetes educational prevention programs and access to medically necessary items. The pervasive lack of knowledge and high costs were found to hamper preventive health behaviors in rural Appalachia.

> *Mrs. Napier has not left her husband's side since his admission. When the doctor stops by to see him, she pulls the doctor aside to suggest that maybe the minister and elders can help convince her husband "that he needs to do the Lord's work and he can't do that unless he is healthy." The doctor says, "I'm not sure that I see the benefit of inviting more people to speak to your husband. Let's see how he feels in a few weeks."*

7   What role, if any, could the minister and elders play in Mr. Napier's care?

As part of a detailed history, it would have been ascertained that Mr. Napier is an elder in the local Disciples of Christ Church. He has been very active in the church for many years, and a visit from the minister and some elders may be helpful, especially if his wife feels that this could motivate him to take better care of himself. In order to better understand the request, the doctor might have asked his wife what would be involved in this visit. Facilitating a visit that would be consistent with the patient's religious beliefs and not be disruptive with the hospital staff would be a valuable goal. Finally, after more discussions, the doctor agrees, and later that evening, the minister and elders from Mr. Napier's church come to visit. The minister explains to Mr. Napier that "a man must accept the law of the Father, the grace of the Spirit, and the mercy of Jesus to have salvation." Although he believes that miracles do occur, and prays for a miracle to cure his diabetes, he also conveys that it is God who has made modern medicine available to us and this medicine may be the miracle. After the visit, Mr. Napier informs the doctor that he is ready to start his prescribed medications.

8   What resources may be available to rural communities to help patients control their diabetes and overcome many of the barriers that exist?

Prior to discussions with Mr. Napier and his family, it is important to identify local county health resources and community intervention programs available to help families in the areas where they live. For example, traveling clinics may be offered by a university hospital. TeleCare, which utilizes communications technologies, especially interactive videoconference systems, connects rural patients and clinicians to the health care resources at a local university medical center. Additionally, recruiting the local clergy to develop a health ministry that includes and have diabetes evaluation could augment current services.

State and federal programs and community consciousness-raising activities can influence development of programs and revenue that will enable diabetic patients, such as Mr. Napier, to become familiar with and able to access diabetic outreach programs that are closer to their home. It is clear that diabetes has reached epidemic proportions, and it is no surprise that in medically underserved rural communities, such as in the Appalachian regions, the need for expansion of diabetes public health programs remains urgently needed. Health care policy must focus on heightening awareness and finding ways to improve access to care, self-management of diabetes, treatment options, and education programs.

Urban vs. Rural Health Care Challenges

The lack of health insurance and not having a usual source of care (i.e. not having a person or place to go to when sick or in need of advice about their health) significantly impacts access to health care for all residents living in the United States. The Agency for Health Care Research and Quality, Medical Expenditure Panel Survey examined variations in the health care expenditures in urban and rural areas between 1998 and 2000. Results showed that, although the proportion of elderly people without Medicare supplemental coverage appears highest in rural counties (38.6%), the difference from metro, near metro, and near rural counties was not significant.

Another study that examined differences among rural, urban, and suburban residents found that rural citizens fared worse than their more urban/suburban counterparts. This study also reported that the most rural and the most urban were found to lack health insurance coverage, when compared with suburban areas. A resident living in the South Bronx, where the percentage of residents living below the poverty level is more than 30% (three times the national average), presents to his or her doctor with a strikingly similar story to Mr. Napier. Lack of insurance may lead to inadequate referrals to a specialist and avoidance of high-cost medications. Even fewer choices exist when trying to adhere to exercise recommendations, such as "go out and take a walk," when personal safety is an issue.

References: Case 25

Astrow AB. Puchalski CM, Sulmasy DP. Religion spirituality, and health care: social, ethical, and practical considerations. *Am J Med* 2001;110:283–7.

Betancourt J.R., Green A.R., Carillo J.E., Ananeh-Firempong O. Defining cultural competency: a practical framework for addressing radical and ethnic disparities on health and healthcare. *Public Health Rep* 2003;118:293–302.

Buryska JF. Assessing the ethical weight of cultural, religious and spiritual claims in the clinical context. *J Med Ethics* 2001;27:118–22.

Cooper L.A., Roter D.L. Patient-provider communication: the effect of race and ethnicity on process and outcomes of healthcare. In: Smedley B.D., Stitch A.M., Nelson A.R., eds. *Unequal Treatment: Confronting Racial and Ethnic Disparities in Healthcare.* The National Academic Press, Washington DC, 2002, pp 552–83.

Eberhardt M.S., Pamuk E.R. The importance of place of residence: examining health in rural and non-rural areas. *Am J Pub Health* 2004;94(10):1682–6.

Indian Health Services. Available at: http://www.ihs.gov.

Kleinman A., Eisenberg L., Good B. Culture, illness and care: clinical lessons from anthropological and cross-cultural research. *Ann Intern Med* 1978; 88:251–88.

Lo B, Kates LW, Ruston D, Arnold RM, Cohen CB, Puchalski CM, Pantilat SZ, Rabow MW, Schreiber RS, Tulsky JA. Responding to requests regarding prayer and religious ceremonies by patients near the end of life and their families. *J Palliat Med* 2003;6:409-415.

Murphy E., Kinmonth A.L. No symptoms, no problems? Patients' understanding of non-insulin diabetes. *Fam Prac* 1995;12:184–92.

Rural Health. Available at: http://www.ruralhealthweb.org.

Sharon L., Larson P.D., Steven R., Machlin A., Nixon M.A., Marc Z. Chartbook #13: healthcare in urban and rural areas, combined years 1998–2000. Agency for Healthcare Research and Quality, Rockville, 2004.

Smith S.L., Tessaro I.A. Cultural perspectives on diabetes in an Appalachian population. *Am J Health Behav* 2005;29(4):291–301.

Tessaro I., Smith S.L., Rye S. Knowledge and perceptions of diabetes in an Appalachian population. *Prev Chron Dis* 2005;2:2;A13.

Zimmerman R. South Bronx environmental studies: public health and environmental policy analysis final report. Institution for Civil Infrastructure Systems 2002;1–135.

APPENDIX 1
Positioning The Interpreter

The following should be done to effectively use an interpreter, particularly when someone other than a trained interpreter is used:

- Have a pre-interview discussion with the interpreter. (Tell the interpreter what you hope to accomplish with this interview and give a brief description of how the patient came to the current situation.)

- Position the interpreter to the side and slightly behind the patient/parent (see Figure).

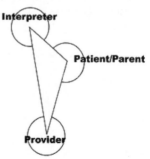

- Look at the patient/parent and not at the interpreter. (Experienced interpreters actually avoid eye contact with everyone in order to promote optimal interaction between the clinician and the parent and/or patient.)

- Speak in short sentences and avoid jargon and phrases that may not translate well from English into another language, such as "the ball is your court."

(It is important to note that interpretation refers to the spoken word, whereas translation is about the written word.)

Source: Horace M. DeLisser, MD, and Lisa Hark, PhD, RD, University of Pennsylvania School of Medicine, 2009. Used with permission

Achieving Cultural Competency: A case-based approach to training health professionals,
1st edition. Edited by L Hark, H DeLisser. © 2009 Blackwell Publishing,
ISBN: 9781405180726.

APPENDIX 2

Kleinman's Explanatory Model of Illness

Kleinman and associates (1978) in their seminal paper further discuss the importance of the explanatory model: "Eliciting the patient's (explanatory) model gives the physician knowledge of the beliefs the patient holds about his illness, the personal and social meaning he attaches to his disorder, his expectations about what will happen to him and what the doctor will do, and his own therapeutic goals. Comparison of patient model with the doctor's model enables the clinician to identify major discrepancies that may cause problems for clinical management. Such comparisons also help the clinician know which aspects of his explanatory model need clearer exposition to patients (and families), and what sort of patient education is most appropriate. And they clarify conflicts not related to different levels of knowledge but different values and interests. Part of the clinical process involves negotiations between these explanatory models, once they have been made explicit."

Eliciting the Patient's Explanatory Model of illness through a set of targeted questions shown below is an important tool for facilitating cross-cultural communication, ensuring patient understanding, and identifying areas of conflict that will need to be negotiated. The wording and number of questions used will vary depending on the characteristics of the patient, the problem, and the setting.

- What do you think has caused your problem?
- Why do you think it started when it did?
- What do you think your sickness does to you? How does it work?
- How severe is your sickness? Will it have a short or long course?
- What kind of treatment do you think you should receive?

Achieving Cultural Competency: A case-based approach to training health professionals, 1st edition. Edited by L Hark, H DeLisser. © 2009 Blackwell Publishing, ISBN: 9781405180726.

- What are the most important results you hope to receive from this treatment?
- What are the chief problems your sickness has caused for you?
- What do you fear most about your sickness?

Adapted from, Kleinman A., Eisenberg L., Good B. Culture, illness, and care: clinical lessons from anthropological and cross-cultural research. *Ann Intern Med* 1978;88:251–88.

Achieving Cultural Competency:
A Case-Based Approach to Training
Health Professionals

Duration: Maximum of 25 hours, each case should take 1 hour
Credit: Up to 25 *AMA PRA Category 1 Credits*™, each case is awarded
1 *AMA PRA Category 1 Credit*™

Original Release Date: June 1, 2009
Last Review Date: January 5, 2009
Expiration: May 31, 2012

Completion Instructions

- To receive CME credit for each case that you complete from this book, please visit the University of Pennsylvania Office of Continuing Medical Education website at: http://www.med.upenn.edu/cme/culture/
- Once on the site, you will be presented with the option to choose from two topics. The topic for this book is called "Achieving Cultural Competency Book Cases (Wiley-Blackwell 2009)". After choosing this topic, you will be presented **with a complete list of cases from this book.**
  Select the case(s) for which you would like to receive CME credit.
- In order to access any of these cases, you must have an account on the CME Website (complementary).
- If you *do not* have an account, sign-up (click on **member sign-up** at the top of the page).
- If you have an account, log into the site with your e-mail address and password (click on **log-in** at the top of the page).
- Next, register for a particular activity (case) by using the link in the "Course Materials" box on the right. When prompted for an access code, enter: **culturebook** (Note: the access code is case-sensitive).
- Click on the "Get CME" link in the "Course Materials" box.
- You now need to complete the Post-Test.
- After successfully completing the Post-Test, with a **score of 75% or higher**, you will be directed to the Evaluation.
- After completing the Evaluation, you will be able to view, print, or save a CME certificate verifying your credit for this activity.

Multiple Choice Questions

Case 1: Ruth Franklin: A 40-year-old African American woman with heart failure

Select the best answer

1 Women from which of the following groups are least likely to perceive themselves as overweight?
   a. African American.
   b. Caucasian.
   c. Asian.
   d. Native American.

2 Which of the following statements best describes the importance of addressing a patient's anger during an office visit?
   a. Eliminates the possibility of a lawsuit against the physician.
   b. Enhances the physician's alliance with the patient.
   c. Prevents the physician from pursuing sensitive issues about the patient.
   d. Establishes the physician's authority over the patient.

3 When a patient expresses anger about a physician's colleague, which of the following statements would be the most appropriate response?
   a. Why are you so aggravated over something so trivial?
   b. Before I ask any questions, please calm down.
   c. What concerns do you have about how you were treated?
   d. Why don't we go talk to Dr. X about your anger?

4 Physicians who provide pharmaceutical samples in their offices should be aware of which of the following statements?
   a. Patients prefer to fill their prescriptions at the pharmacy rather than receive samples.
   b. It is standard practice to give out free samples in physicians' offices.
   c. Prescriptions written by physicians are typically not influenced by office samples.
   d. There may be a significant price difference between samples and the generic version of the medication.

5 How should physicians and office staff respond to patients who chronically miss appointments?

   a. Assume the patient does not want treatment and ask him/her to change doctors.

   b. Bill the patient for the missed appointment when he/she is a "no show."

   c. Speak directly to the patient about the missed appointments.

   d. Accuse the patient of being insensitive and taking up valuable time.

6 In what context is it appropriate to use pejorative phrases when describing patients?

   a. It is never acceptable to use pejorative phrases to describe patients.

   b. In the presence of the patient.

   c. Privately, with staff or other hospital employees.

   d. Only in the presence of a trusted colleague.

7 How should a health professional approach a colleague about his/her culturally insensitive behavior or remarks?

   a. He/She should be tolerant and open to the colleague's opinions.

   b. He/She should avoid direct confrontation with the colleague.

   c. He/She should warn other patients about the colleague.

   d. He/She should speak honestly, but respectfully, to the colleague.

8 Health disparities have been shown to exist in regard to organ transplantation. African American and Hispanic patients may encounter which of the following compared with their non-Hispanic white counterparts?

   a. Shorter time in getting referred to a transplant specialist.

   b. Shorter time on the organ transplant list.

   c. Lower rates of graft survival after receiving an organ transplant.

   d. Lower mortality after receiving an organ transplant.

Case 2: Carl Jones: A 48-year-old homeless Caucasian man with chest pain and lung cancer

Select the best answer

1 Which of the following factors may contribute to the higher mortality rates seen in the homeless population?
   a. Increased exposure to air pollution.
   b. Overprescription of psychotropic medications.
   c. Suboptimal access to health care.
   d. Stress-induced high blood pressure.

2 What approach should physicians use in taking care of uncooperative, self-abusing, or disruptive patients from a low socioeconomic group?
   a. Establish authority in the patient–doctor relationship by using stern language.
   b. Refrain from following up on such patients when possible.
   c. Ensure that personal biases do not taint clinical judgment.
   d. Allow patients' self-destructive behaviors to subside before administering treatment.

3 How should physicians treat patients who they suspect are incapable of keeping follow-up appointments?
   a. Encourage patients to educate themselves and take responsibility for their health.
   b. Establish a system of penalties to increase retention rate.
   c. Disregard patients' incapacities and fit them into the schedule.
   d. Discuss the importance of personal responsibility before administering follow-up care.

4 Poor adherence results in which of the following outcomes?
   a. Increased patient morbidities and mortalities.
   b. Slight improvement in health.
   c. Reduced health care costs.
   d. Weakened physician–patient relationship.

5 Which of the following physician barriers can affect a patient's adherence?
   a. Lack of insight into the patient's illness.
   b. Inadequate explanation of instructions.
   c. Cost of medications or treatment.
   d. Distraction by other life issues or priorities.

6 Which of the following health care system barriers can affect a patient's adherence?
   a. Treatment of asymptomatic disease.
   b. Inadequate follow-up or discharge planning.
   c. Forgetfulness.
   d. Inadequate health insurance.

7 How should physicians respond to working professionals, in comparison to unemployed or low-income patients?
   a. Physicians should be more flexible with scheduling low-income patients.
   b. Patients from professional occupations should be afforded greater respect.
   c. Physicians should promote patients' health regardless of their socioeconomic status.
   d. Physicians should fulfill the requests of other working professionals without hesitation.

8 How might the perspectives of financially secure patients with respect to end-of-life care differ from those of disadvantaged patients?
   a. Financially secure patients are more likely to insist that everything be done to keep them alive.
   b. Disadvantaged patients may interpret end-of-life care as an attempt to deny essential treatments.
   c. Disadvantaged patients are more likely to want to spend their last days outside the hospital.
   d. Financially secure patients are more likely to demand placement in assisted living facilities to avoid burdening their families.

Case 3: Maria Morales: A 57-year-old Mexican woman with type 2 diabetes

Select the best answer

1 Which of the following approaches is most effective in helping patients with type 2 diabetes to lose weight?
   a. Advocate the American Diabetes Association's 1800-calorie diet for all patients.
   b. Recommend daily exercise and decreased food intake.
   c. Suggest substituting healthy ingredients for meals and snacks based on the patient's cultural heritage and personal preferences.
   d. Refer patients to a dietitian for all their diet-related inquiries.

2 From which of the following ethnic backgrounds are patients most likely to change their diet after being diagnosed with a health problem by their physician?
  a. Asian.
  b. Latino/Hispanic.
  c. African American.
  d. Caucasian.

3 Many Latino patients incorrectly associate diabetes with which of the following symptoms?
  a. Malnutrition.
  b. Overexertion.
  c. Vitamin overdose.
  d. Depression.

4 How should physicians approach patients with type 2 diabetes patients who also regularly visit holistic healers (*curanderos*)?
  a. Take a history of alternative medicines used by patients to avoid herb–drug interactions.
  b. Highlight the shortcomings of herbal remedies for treating type 2 diabetes.
  c. Meet with the holistic healer to discuss the patient's diabetes.
  d. Disregard the patient's use of alternative medicines.

5 Among Latino patients with diabetes, which of the following factors is most important in determining adherence to medication and instilling self-confidence?
  a. Physician support.
  b. Establishing a daily routine.
  c. Family support.
  d. Eliciting the Patient's Explanatory Model.

6 Which of the following is the best approach when referring a Mexican patient with type 2 diabetes to a dietitian for medical nutrition therapy?
  a. Make the referral as quickly as possible.
  b. Attempt to identify a bilingual dietitian familiar with the Mexican diet.
  c. Assume the dietitian is knowledgeable about all aspects of the Mexican diet.
  d. Meet with the dietitian on a regular basis to keep up with the patient's eating habits.

7 When encountering patients with misconceptions regarding insulin therapy for diabetes, how should the physician respond?
   a. Agree with the patient about insulin.
   b. Reject patients' misconceptions directly.
   c. Assure patients that their fears are based more on superstition than fact.
   d. Clarify the role of insulin by highlighting cause and effect.

8 How should health professionals respond to the widened definitions of prediabetes and diabetes by the World Health Organization, the American Diabetes Association, and other organizations?
   a. Assist patients in identifying evidence-based health care resources.
   b. Recommend that patients do their own diabetes research online.
   c. Expect to diagnose fewer patients with prediabetes.
   d. Make no major changes in clinical practice.

Case 4: Maya Mohammed: 15-year-old Arab American teenager with leukemia

Select the best answer

1 When is it appropriate to ask a Muslim patient about his/her sexual activity?
   a. Only if the patient is over 18 years old.
   b. Only in a sensitive manner when it is relevant to the care of the patient.
   c. It is not appropriate to ask a Muslim patient about his/her sexual history directly.
   d. Only if the patient is married.

2 Prior to the physical examination of a Muslim adolescent patient, which of the following statements should be clarified to the patient and his/her parent?
   a. The examination is not critical to the patient's immediate treatment.
   b. Proper draping is optional for the examination.
   c. The parent may not be in the room with the patient during the examination.
   d. They can express concerns about any part of the exam at any time.

3 In Arab culture and Islam, which of the following parties may participate in medically related decisions for an adolescent patient?
   a. Senior family members.
   b. The patient's father.
   c. The individual patient.
   d. All of the above.

4 When preparing to examine a Muslim woman or girl, it is appropriate to request that she do which of the following?
   a. Remove her clothes, including her hijab, and put on a gown and drape.
   b. Keep on all of her clothes, including her hijab.
   c. Remove only those clothes that relate to the presenting complaint.
   d. Remove her clothes, keeping on the hijab if she prefers, and put on a gown and drape.

5 Which of the following factors might lead the parents of a Muslim or Arab adolescent patient to initially delay or refuse chemotherapy?
   a. Belief related to Islam.
   b. Superstitions about chemotherapy in Arab culture.
   c. Desire to consult with extended family members and/or Imam first.
   d. Higher prevalence of chemotherapy-related complications among Arabs.

6 Which of the following groups are not required to fast during Ramadan, a major Muslim religious observance?
   a. Anyone who is sick.
   b. Medical students.
   c. Adolescents.
   d. Adult women.

7 When communicating with a Muslim patient about end-of-life issues, which of the following statements best shows respect and mindfulness about Muslim beliefs?
   a. Death is expected soon.
   b. We are fighting a losing battle.
   c. We need to start considering options for hospice care.
   d. No one knows when, where, or how someone will die.

8 Which of the following services would be especially helpful for terminally ill Muslim patients?

a. Referring the patient for additional tests.

b. Negotiating a plan for outside visitors, especially the Imam.

c. Providing patients with motivational pamphlets.

d. Serving regular hospital meals.

Case 5: Jon Le: A 48-year-old Korean man with cerebral hemorrhage

Select the best answer

1 Moxibustion (or moxa), through heat generated by the burning of mugwort (a spongy herb), is used by traditional Chinese practitioners to treat many conditions. Which of the following Western treatments is most likely to be impacted by concurrent moxibustion?

a. Oral medications.

b. Topical medications.

c. Inhaled medications.

d. Surgical interventions.

2 Which of the following statements is true about the nature of acculturation?

a. High levels lead to better health.

b. Lower levels lead to better health.

c. Differing patterns within families may lead to intergenerational conflict.

d. Levels are influenced mostly by length of time in the U.S.

3 Assimilationists, separationists, and integrationists characterize which model of acculturation?

a. Multidimensional.

b. Bidimensional.

c. Tridimensional.

d. Unidimensional.

4 Which of the following groups describes the majority of users of complementary and alternative medicine in the U.S.?

a. Poorly educated Chinese Americans.

b. Highly educated Caucasians.

c. Highly educated African Americans.

d. Poorly educated Korean Americans.

5 When approaching patients about their use of complementary and alternative medicine (CAM), what is the physician's primary objective?
   a. To discourage patients from seeing CAM healthcare providers.
   b. To promote the patient's adherence to prescribed medication in addition to CAM.
   c. To establish an open discussion about all aspects of the patient's health care.
   d. To gradually dissuade patients from using CAM.

6 Which of the following questions is most effective in identifying a patient's ethnicity?
   a. Do you consider yourself Asian?
   b. Are you Chinese?
   c. When did you first come to the U.S.?
   d. What ethnic identity best describes you?

7 The LEARN acronym is a useful tool for treating patients from diverse backgrounds. What does the "A" stand for?
   a. Acknowledge and discuss differences and similarities.
   b. Admit personal shortcomings regarding patients' cultural backgrounds.
   c. Advocate treatment.
   d. Argue for medical perceptions and understandings of the problem.

8 Which of the following questions can be used to initiate the process of "LEARNing?"
   a. When can I see you again?
   b. What do you think your sickness does to you?
   c. Have you been taking your medication?
   d. When was the last time you came in?

Case 6: Nadia Rosenberg: A 53-year-old Russian woman with drug-resistant tuberculosis

Select the best answer

1 Physicians encounter many patients who may be unaccustomed to the U.S. health care system. How can physicians effectively take care of patients from diverse backgrounds?
   a. Physicians should focus on their communication skills over understanding a patient's cultural context.
   b. Physicians should emphasize good communication in combination with understanding a patient's cultural context.
   c. Physicians should prioritize understanding a patient's cultural context and leave communication to a trained medical interpreter.
   d. Physicians should treat all patients in the same manner, regardless of a patient's preconceived notions of the U.S. health care system.

2 Language is an unavoidable barrier for many patients in the U.S. What role do ad hoc interpreters play in bridging the language gap?
   a. Ad hoc interpreters may be helpful, but they lack the clinical foundation and experience of trained medical interpreters.
   b. Ad hoc interpreters make invaluable contributions to patient care.
   c. Ad hoc interpreters are economical and convenient for physicians and patients.
   d. Ad hoc interpreters offer little help in communicating with patients.

3 Which of the following skills do trained medical interpreters provide in the clinical setting?
   a. They can help the patient make health care decisions.
   b. They are generally proficient in explaining clinical terminology to patients in an understandable cultural context and with limited distortion.
   c. They have an extensive knowledge of the patient's medical history.
   d. They provide the social and spontaneous interactions with patients, such as "small talk" for the development of rapport.

4 When employing a trained medical interpreter, which of the following is the ideal sitting position relative to the doctor and the patient?

   a. The interpreter should sit next to, and slightly behind the physician and make eye contact with the patient.

   b. The interpreter should sit between the patient and the physician to emphasize the facilitator role and avoid making eye contact with both parties.

   c. The interpreter should sit next to the patient and make eye contact with the physician.

   d. The interpreter should sit next to, and slightly behind the patient and avoid eye contact with the physician.

5 A trusting physician–patient relationship is a key factor in improving patient adherence to prescribed medications. Which of the following might discourage a patient from taking his/her medications?

   a. Using a trained medical interpreter to explain a prescription schedule.

   b. Discussing folk or culture beliefs in the context of treating illness.

   c. Prescribing complex treatments.

   d. Reinforcing the urgency of the patient's illness.

6 Which of the following questions is an effective way to elicit a Patient's explanatory model of illness regarding tuberculosis symptoms?

   a. What is your understanding of tuberculosis?

   b. How long have you had tuberculosis?

   c. Does your family have a history of tuberculosis?
     Have you ever been tested for tuberculosis?

7 Direct observed treatment (DOT) is the appropriate treatment for patients with multi-drug-resistant tuberculosis. What is the best approach for physicians to initially take when a patient requires DOT?

   a. Immediately initiate DOT when the patient's diagnosis is confirmed.

   b. Ensure the patient understands the diagnosis, the importance of the treatment, and how this will impact his/her life.

   c. Alert the patient's family, friends, and coworkers of the elevated risk of tuberculosis infection.

   d. Give the patient time to consider whether the DOT is within his/her budget.

8 Why might an immigrant patient be reluctant to participate in DOT?
   a. Immigrant patients are fearful of medical authority.
   b. The patient may be fearful because of the loss of privacy or cultural misunderstanding.
   c. The patient may have had a similar experience in his/her native country.
   d. The patient may feel that DOT will make the illness worse.

9 Under what conditions is the DOT program most successful?
   a. When DOT is carried out in a way that is convenient for a patient to enable completion of the recommended therapy.
   b. When DOT is monitored directly by an attending physician at a local health center.
   c. When DOT is only administered when the patient's symptoms of illness are most severe, based on the patient's wishes.
   d. When DOT is administered when the patient cooperates with hospital instructions.

Case 7: Isabel Delgado: A 47-year-old Dominican woman with hypertension

Select the best answer

1 Which of the following is most likely to improve a patient's adherence to taking medications?
   a. Providing free samples in the office.
   b. Creating a system of punishments for nonadherent patients.
   c. Discussing alternative therapies with patients.
   d. Having continuity of care during office visits.

2 Which of the following is likely to be an important benefit of exploring a Patient's Explanatory Model of Illness?
   a. Improved patient adherence and increased understanding of the patient's perspective.
   b. Less complaints about the physician from the patient.
   c. Prompt payment of physician fees.
   d. Less litigation.

3 Which of the following statements is correct regarding family and friends' influence on a patient's medication choices?

a. Family and friends tend to support the physician's medication recommendations.

b. Family and friends may offer medical advice that contradicts the physician's advice.

c. Family and friends rarely influence a patient's medication choices.

d. It is difficult to quantify how family and friends influence a patient's medication choices.

4 Which of the following questions may help identify social factors that would impact a patient's adherence?

a. Do you ever consume alternative medications?

b. Do you remember the last time you took your medications?

c. Aside from your health, what else in your life is worrying you?

d. Why wouldn't you want to take your medication?

5 Which of the following is an effective approach to prescribing medications for patients from diverse cultural backgrounds?

a. Work with a nontraditional healer.

b. Admonish patients who rely only on alternative medicine.

c. Remind patients of the universal efficacy of Western medicine.

d. Learn about culturally relevant medicinal practices of patients before prescribing medication.

6 Patients who are very deferential toward physicians may respond in which of the following ways when prescribed medication?

a. Inquire about the medical cost.

b. Avoid asking about side effects.

c. Document their medication intake.

d. Ask how the medicine works.

7 ETHNIC is a framework for culturally competent clinical practice. Which of the following choices is not a component of this acronym?

a. Explanation.

b. Healers.

c. Interpretation.

d. Collaboration.

8 Which of the following questions is taken from the "Treatment" component of the ETHNIC acronym?

    a. Do you know anyone else who has had the symptoms you are experiencing?

    b. Is there anything you eat, drink, or do on a regular basis to stay healthy?

    c. Have you sought advice from an alternative medicine practitioner?

    d. What are the most important results you hope to achieve by using this treatment?

Case 8: George Dennis: A 35-year-old African American man with AIDS

Select the best answer

1 Why might a patient be reluctant to reveal his/her sexual orientation to a health care provider?

    a. The patient may not self-identify as gay.

    b. Uncertainty about how this health care provider will react.

    c. Fear of being stereotyped or stigmatized.

    d. All of the above.

2 When taking a medical history, which of the following approaches would be the best way to develop a patient's trust and build rapport?

    a. Confront a patient with targeted questions about his/her behaviors in a direct manner.

    b. Provide a setting that is private and safe for disclosure.

    c. Always include family members in these conversations.

    d. Be persistent in your questioning of the patient.

3 When questioning a male patient about his sexual orientation, which of the following statements would be most appropriate?

    a. Are you gay?

    b. Would you consider yourself a homosexual?

    c. Are you sexually active with other men?

    d. Do you sleep with men?

4 When discussing sensitive and personal issues with a patient that may involve significant lifestyle changes and treatment issues, how should the patient's family be involved in this process?

   a. The patient's family should always be actively involved in the conversation.

   b. The patient's family is not an important participant in the conversation.

   c. The physician should always decide whether or not to include the family based on the patient's wishes.

   d. The physician should contact the family prior to speaking with the patient.

5 Which of the following statements is correct regarding identifying patients at risk for HIV infection?

   a. All patients should be considered as being at risk for HIV infection.

   b. Only homosexual patients should be considered at risk for HIV infection.

   c. Only patients who use intravenous drugs should be considered at risk for HIV infection.

   d. A monogamous heterosexual woman is not considered at risk for HIV infection.

6 If it is the right of the patient to decide whom to disclose personal medical information to, how should the physician respond when requested to withhold information about a diagnosis from family members?

   a. Attempt to convince the patient to tell his/her family of their diagnosis.

   b. Ignore the patient's request and ask to have a family conference.

   c. Accept the patient's wishes without further discussion.

   d. Initiate further discussion and help the patient identify a surrogate decision maker.

7 What is the role of the physician when the patient lacks decision-making capacity and someone other than a family member has been designated as the surrogate decision maker?

   a. Follow the instructions of the family and ignore the surrogate.

   b. Ignore the family and talk only to the surrogate.

   c. Serve as a mediator between parties and encourage all groups to work together in the best interest of the patient, consistent with the patient's wishes.

   d. Consult legal affairs to determine who should be the decision-maker.

8 Which of the following correctly identifies the role of the physician and the patient in making health care decisions?

   a. The physician is the ultimate authority in making decisions about a patient's health.

   b. The physician and the patient must establish together who makes decisions about the patient's health.

   c. The physician has little direct influence on the patient's personal health choices.

   d. Although it is the physician's responsibility to instruct the patient about his or her condition, the physician must ultimately respect the patient's personal health choices.

Case 9: Mary Jones: A 2-year-old Caucasian girl with delayed speech development

Select the best answer

1 Which of the following approaches may aid a health care provider in understanding the factors that affect adherence?

   a. Schedule monthly follow-up appointments.

   b. Ask patients if they understand how to take their medications.

   c. Find out the significant sources of stress in patients' lives.

   d. Offer liquid or chewable alternatives to medicine that must be swallowed.

2 Which of the following choices constitutes one of the four domains of the "social context review of systems"?

   a. Lifestyle.

   b. Self-esteem.

   c. Family.

   d. Change of environment.

3 Which of the following questions is associated directly with the domain of life control?

   a. How do you deal with the stress in your life?

   b. Do you ever feel that you are treated unfairly by the health care system?

   c. Do you have trouble reading the instructions on your medicine bottles?

   d. Do you feel that God (or spirituality) provides a strong source of support in your life?

4 What is the primary purpose of the Transtheoretical Model as adapted for this case study?
  a. To identify where the patient is in his/her thinking.
  b. To correct the patient's misunderstanding of prescription instructions.
  c. To improve patient retention rates.
  d. To elicit the Patient's Explanatory Model.

5 Low health literacy is associated with which of the following outcomes?
  a. Better communication with providers.
  b. Increased hospitalizations.
  c. Increased medical adherence.
  d. High retention rates.

6 Which of the following approaches may lead to increased levels of patient understanding?
  a. Providing medical pamphlets.
  b. Giving verbal instructions for taking medications.
  c. Having the patient restate in his/her own words the directions that have just been given.
  d. Explaining how to use several different medications during the same session.

7 Rates of illiteracy can often be determined based on which of the following criteria?
  a. U.S. citizenship.
  b. Age.
  c. Socioeconomic status.
  d. None of the above.

8 Which of the following choices is an indicator of low literacy level?
  a. Questioning the medication dose on a label.
  b. Incomplete health questionnaires.
  c. Inadequate follow-up for scheduled appointments.
  d. Having an illiterate spouse.

9 Which of the following choices is an effective complement to motivational interviewing?
  a. Using confidence and importance rating scales.
  b. Arranging group motivational meetings with other patients.
  c. Referring patients to a social worker.
  d. Spending time to recall personal experience.

Case 10: Priya Krishnamurthy: A 73-year-old South Asian Indian woman with a stroke

Select the best answer

1 When treating a patient who cannot speak English, what is the primary advantage of using a professional medical interpreter instead of family members?
   a. Professional interpreters always have more medical knowledge than family members.
   b. Professional interpreters can calm emotionally distressed patients.
   c. Professional interpreters can offer direct interpretation of the patient's responses.
   d. Professional interpreters always have a better command of the English language.

2 Which of the following is a true statement regarding the adjustment process during the acculturation?
   a. Age has no effect on the adjustment process.
   b. Older adults tend to experience greater difficulty adjusting to a new culture.
   c. Individuals who immigrated early in life have more trouble adjusting.
   d. Individuals who immigrated late in life are generally more willing to adjust.

3 Which mode of decisionmaking is prevalent among families of Asian Indian origin?
   a. Individual deliberation.
   b. Conscious belief-based deliberation.
   c. Instinct-based deliberation.
   d. Communal deliberation.

4 Which of the following may be the most effective approach to ensure good communication with a large family of a hospitalized patient?
   a. Ask the family to choose an individual to be the point of contact with the health care team.
   b. Appoint the person who spends the most time at the patient's bedside to be the point of contact with the health care team.
   c. Listen to each family member's individual concerns.
   d. Arrange a daily meeting with the entire family to discuss the patient's health care.

5 Which of the following is an effective way to address cultural issues about personal contact in a clinical care setting?
   a. Be considerate of the patient's requests not to be touched.
   b. Attempt to accommodate the patient's requests whenever possible, while providing medically appropriate care.
   c. Identify a chaperone and override the patient's requests in order to expedite their care.
   d. Ask that a family member remain at the bedside at all times to oversee patient care.

6 When diet is affected by cultural factors, which in turn significantly impact a patient's health care, which of the following approaches is appropriate?
   a. Recommend immediate cessation of the usual diet and provide a list of prohibited foods.
   b. Allow the patient to continue his/her usual diet and adjust medications accordingly.
   c. Discuss the underlying cultural factors related to the usual diet and explore options within that paradigm that might be better suited to the patient's health.
   d. Suggest that the patient instead see a physician who shares his/her cultural background.

7 Patients of Asian Indian origin who use alternative medical treatments are most likely to subscribe to which of the following?
   a. Moxibustion.
   b. Reiki.
   c. Ayurvedic medicine.
   d. Opium.

8 When a patient requires long-term care, which of the following issues must be addressed by the family and the health care providers?
   a. How the family expects to manage the patient's finances.
   b. How the patient and family feel about nursing homes.
   c. Which nursing home has doctors or nurses with the same cultural background.
   d. Which family member will tell the patient that he/she cannot return home.

9 Cultural and religious issues may impact which of the following issues related to end-of-life care?

    a. Creating an advance directive.

    b. Using a feeding tube.

    c. Using medication for pain control.

    d. All of the above.

Case 11: Carlos Cruz: A 34-year-old Mexican man with sleep apnea and metabolic syndrome

Select the best answer

1 When a health care provider believes that there is a language barrier with a patient over the phone, what is the best course of action?

    a. If available, ask a bilingual staff member to join the conversation.

    b. If available, have a bilingual staff member take over the conversation.

    c. Inform the patient that there is an obvious language barrier.

    d. Request that the patient come into the office to meet in person.

2 How should a health care provider respond to a colleague's complaints about a patient that might reflect ethnic insensitivity?

    a. Understand that the colleague's complaints are to be expected and don't respond.

    b. Emphasize the primary importance of compassion toward patients.

    c. Chastise the colleague for expressing personal bias.

    d. Sympathize with the colleague's complaints and draw from personal experience.

3 Which of the following factors play the largest role in determining a patient's explanatory model?

    a. Medical history.

    b. Education level.

    c. Family background.

    d. Culture.

4 The prevalence of sleep apnea, and its association with obesity, is greater among which of the following groups?

    a. African Americans and Caucasians.

    b. Caucasians and Native Americans.

    c. Native Americans and Hispanics.

    d. Hispanics and Asian Americans.

5 After ensuring the patient understands the nature of sleep apnea and how to use the CPAP machine, which of the following measures would be effective in improving low CPAP adherence?
   a. Contact family members and loved ones to encourage patient adherence.
   b. Discuss barriers that the patient has encountered when using the device.
   c. Start the patient on a mild sedative to be taken nightly.
   d. Enroll the patient in a sleep study to monitor CPAP usage.

6 Sleep apnea is most dangerous among individuals from which of the following occupations?
   a. Construction.
   b. Military.
   c. Farming.
   d. Truck driving.

7 The greatest health benefits occur when sedentary individuals incorporate which of the following levels of exercise as part of their lifestyle?
   a. All levels of exercise offer similar benefit, as long as they are carried out daily.
   b. Low-intensity exercise.
   c. Moderate-intensity exercise.
   d. High-intensity exercise.

8 Which of the following statements is more likely to convince a truck driver to change his behavior and eat more healthy foods?
   a. You should refuel your body just as you refuel your truck, with healthy foods.
   b. You should eat nine fruits and vegetables daily to decrease constipation.
   c. You should decrease your caloric intake because you eat too much.
   d. You should drink a lot more water, at least 10 cups every day.

Case 12: Denise Smith: A 41-year-old Caucasian woman with asthma

Select the best answer

1 Which of the following groups have been referred to as an "invisible minority" within the health care system?
   a. Lesbians.
   b. Illegal immigrants.
   c. Muslims.
   d. Native Americans.

2 When meeting an androgynous-appearing patient for the first time, what is the best approach?
   a. Assume that the patient is homosexual and begin by taking her medical history.
   b. Ask the patient if she is a lesbian upon introducing oneself.
   c. Refer to the patient by full name, rather than using an engendered prefix.
   d. Avoid discussing the patient's gender or sexual preferences.

3 How can physicians promote an inclusive medical environment and prevent presumed heterosexism?
   a. Have patients fill out questionnaires with boxes labeled "homosexual."
   b. Open the conversation with a personal anecdote.
   c. Assume all androgynous-appearing patients are gay or bisexual.
   d. Openly discuss sexual history and relationship status with patients.

4 Which of the following choices correctly groups the three components that determine sexual orientation?
   a. Attraction, self-esteem, and ego.
   b. Attraction, cognition, and behavior.
   c. Cognition, behavior, and ego.
   d. Cognition, self-esteem, and behavior.

5 Which of the following barriers to health care may have created health disparities for lesbians in the U.S.?
   a. Homophobia.
   b. Lack of insurance.
   c. Socioeconomic level.
   d. Level of education.

6 Which of the following may make it more difficult for a lesbian woman to quit smoking?
a. Higher rates of schizophrenia.
b. Nicotine is more addicting for women.
c. Targeting of LGBT community members by tobacco companies.
d. Fear of losing weight.

7 What is the primary result of a patient feeling "judged"?
a. The physician and/or the hospital becomes at risk for legal repercussions.
b. The physician's reputation becomes affected.
c. The patient will refuse copayment.
d. The effectiveness of the doctor–patient relationship may be jeopardized.

8 When motivating patients to quit smoking, which of the following approaches is the *most* effective?
a. Direct all patients to a smoking cessation support group.
b. Support each patient's small steps and develop a long-term quitting plan.
c. Provide patients with ample brochures about the dangers of smoking.
d. Remind patients that smoking will kill them in time.

Case 13: Mae Ling Chung: A 22-year-old Chinese woman in an arranged marriage

Select the best answer

1 Which of the following statements is true about marriage in China?
a. Arranged marriages are mostly limited to urban centers.
b. The government only recognizes arranged marriages under law.
c. Free-choice marriage is a right for women age 20 and older.
d. Only one party needs to give consent to an arranged marriage.

2 Studies show that victims of abuse who do not have access to contraception have high rates of which of the following?
a. Unplanned pregnancies that result in terminations.
b. Psychological disorders.
c. Syphilis.
d. Gonorrhea.

3 When domestic violence is suspected in an arranged marriage, the physician should take which of the following approaches to address the issue?

   a. Refer the couple to a culturally appropriate social worker.
   b. Explore the patient's inner thoughts and feelings or partner behavior that might indicate ongoing abuse.
   c. Immediately file a police report against the abuser.
   d. Voice the concern directly in the presence of both parties.

4 Which of the following approaches is effective in building patient trust?

   a. Repeating prescription instructions.
   b. Offering to schedule a follow-up appointment.
   c. Providing written instructions for medications.
   d. Making eye contact with the patient during a visit.

5 When is it appropriate to prescribe birth control pills for a patient in an arranged marriage?

   a. When the patient is experiencing domestic abuse.
   b. When the patient is afraid of getting an STD.
   c. When the patient expresses the desire to not become pregnant.
   d. When the patient appears healthy enough for sexual activity.

6 A complete discussion of contraception should include which of the following?

   a. Verbal explanation of pros and cons for each method.
   b. Verbal and written descriptions of methods.
   c. An opportunity for questions about how each method works.
   d. All of the above.

7 To provide care for a Chinese patient struggling with becoming " *xianqi liangmu,*" which of the following approaches would be the most effective?

   a. Prescribe an antidepressant medication.
   b. Consider referral to a Chinese social worker.
   c. Focus on her immediate health concerns.
   d. Suggest that the patient discuss her concerns with her family.

8 How might physicians who see both partners of an arranged marriage provide culturally sensitive care to both of them?

   a. Recommend a form of contraception that both parties agree on.
   b. Discuss perceived family pressures with each party separately, and then together.
   c. Explain the implications of *"cheng jia li ye"* in U.S. culture.
   d. Refer one party to another physician to minimize bias.

Case 14: Earl Collins: A 73-year-old African American man with lung cancer

Select the best answer

1 Which of the following approaches is an effective way for physicians to address folk beliefs of their patients?
   a. Respectfully dismiss their beliefs as superstitions.
   b. Assure patients that allopathic medicine provides better results than alternative treatments.
   c. Engage patients in discussions about their beliefs while advocating for the treatment that is believed to be the most appropriate.
   d. Demonstrate complete acceptance of the patient's belief.

2 A patient in need of surgery expresses the belief that exposing lung cancer to air during surgery can cause the tumor to spread. What might this belief reflect?
   a. Personal investigation of the mechanisms of cancer spread.
   b. General fear of surgery or distrust of the physician.
   c. A trust in conventional chemotherapy over surgical treatments.
   d. An understanding of the risks and benefits of surgery.

3 The belief stated in the previous question is more common among which of the following ethnic groups?
   a. Hispanic.
   b. Caucasian.
   c. Asian.
   d. African American.

4 A patient is curious about Reiki, a Japanese spiritual practice often used as a complementary therapy. Reiki falls under which category of complementary and alternative medicine?
   a. Manipulative and body-based methods.
   b. Alternative medical systems.
   c. Energy therapies.
   d. Mind–body medicine.

5 How should physicians initiate conversations with patients who use complementary or alternative therapies?
   a. In a frank but open manner.
   b. In a nonjudgmental manner.
   c. In a suspicious manner.
   d. In a curious manner.

6 Which of the following guidelines for the use of nonconventional modalities is correct?
   a. Health care providers should make every attempt to ascertain alternative therapy use during each visit.
   b. All "natural" products are generally safe.
   c. Health care providers should support all alternative therapies.
   d. When using alternative medicines, more is always better than less.

7 When treating life-threatening illnesses, how should physicians respond to the religious beliefs of their patients?
   a. Always give treatment that preserves life and offers the best outcome.
   b. Initiate a respectful discussion that includes the patients' families and/or the patients' spiritual advisors.
   c. Allow the patients to make the appropriate choices excluding outside influences.
   d. Discourage the patients from making a decision based only on their religious beliefs.

Case 15: Irma Matos: A 66-year-old Ecuadorian woman with type 2 diabetes and hypertension

Select the best answer

1 How accessible and regulated are doctor visits and diagnostic testing for patients in Latin America compared with the U.S.?
   a. Very accessible and relatively unregulated.
   b. Very accessible and strictly regulated.
   c. Relatively accessible and regulated.
   d. Inaccessible and unregulated.

2 It is common for Latin American patients with "dual residency" to spend which of the following seasons in their native country?
   a. Fall.
   b. Winter.
   c. Spring.
   d. Summer.

3 Prior to a diabetic patient's extended overseas vacation, which of the following questions about traveling must be asked?
   a. Will you be staying in the city or in the countryside?
   b. What is the climate like there during this time of year?
   c. When was the last time you visited your home country?
   d. Do you have a primary care doctor in your home country for an emergency?

4 When a patient is on vacation, Medicare/Medicaid will provide medication for how many days?
a. 30 days, once per year.
b. 30 days, twice per year.
c. 60 days, once per year.
d. 60 days, twice per year.

5 What is the appeal of "policlinics" in some parts of Ecuador?
a. Local physicians offer free service and medication samples on policlinic days.
b. Policlinics offer inexpensive "general prevention packages," which include a variety of health tests.
c. Patients may visit doctors of multiple specialties at the same time.
d. Policlinics are more sanitary than most public health care clinics.

6 When patients go on vacation, which of the following behaviors is most likely to occur?
a. Forgetting medication instructions.
b. Poor fluid intake.
c. Lack of physical activity.
d. Overconsumption of calories.

7 Which of the following statements about health care in Ecuador and other Latin American countries is true?
a. Pharmacists may give medical treatment without a physician's prescription.
b. Sharing medication among family members is rare in Latin American countries.
c. Few drugs are dispensed without medical prescriptions.
d. Choosing medications is usually left up to the individual.

8 A physician should plan a process for obtaining medication refills if his/her patient is expected to be on vacation for at least how many days?
a. 15 days.
b. 30 days.
c. 60 days.
d. 120 days.

Case 16: Eileen Clark: An 82-year-old African American woman with a stroke

Select the best answer

1 The disproportionate under representation of which of the following ethnic groups in current clinical research may contribute to health-related disparities?
   a. African Americans.
   b. Asian Americans.
   c. Hispanics.
   d. Native Americans.

2 In the context of biomedical research, informed consent should be obtained in which of the following ways?
   a. By any means possible.
   b. By subtle manipulation, if necessary.
   c. In a noncoercive manner.
   d. In a way that maximizes physician control.

3 The Tuskegee Syphilis Study has had which of the following effects on the African American community?
   a. Greater suspicion and reluctance about participating in research studies.
   b. Less use of complementary or alternative medical treatments.
   c. Greater compliance with prescription medications.
   d. Increased testing for syphilis and other sexually transmitted diseases.

4 Which of the following approaches is most likely to address patients' and families' concerns about perceived racial disparities in clinical care and research?
   a. Emphasize that race has no bearing on health care.
   b. Assure patients that all medications and treatments have established safety and efficacy in all race/ethnic groups.
   c. Openly discuss established differences among race/ethnic groups related to treatment and areas where differences may exist but remain unknown.
   d. Limit opportunities for patients to speak to family members and friends about their concerns.

5 Which of the following methods is most effective when getting a consensus among family members of a patient who lacks decision-making capacity?
   a. Remove oneself from the room and allow the family to discuss among themselves.
   b. Tactfully argue for the most effective procedure.
   c. Use active listening to query about decision-making processes, expectations, and understanding of the patient's illness.
   d. Ask the most senior member of the family to make the final decision.

6 How may a physician maintain rapport with a patient and his/her family after gaining their consent?
   a. Provide information about a patient's status when convenient.
   b. Alternate with a qualified nurse in seeing the patient and family.
   c. Always use proper medical jargon to reflect personal proficiency.
   d. Set goals that focus on the patient and are understandable to the family.

Case 17: Leslie O'Malley: A 66-year-old Irish American man with breast cancer

Select the best answer

1 Which of the following statements about drinking patterns in Irish immigrants is true?
   a. Irish immigrants are no more likely to consume alcohol than indigenous groups.
   b. Irish immigrants drink more frequently than all other groups.
   c. Irish immigrants have better tolerance than all other groups.
   d. Irish immigrants are more likely to binge-drink than most other groups.

2 When questioning a patient about his/her alcohol intake, which of the following approaches is most effective?
   a. Frame the question in terms of the patient's ethnicity.
   b. Explain that these questions are always part of a routine social history.
   c. Joke with the patient about your own alcohol intake.
   d. Tell the patient that alcohol is part of everyday life.

3 How might the effect of a diagnosis of breast cancer differ between a woman and a man?

   a. A male patient may be more concerned about his personal survival.

   b. A male patient may fear disfiguring surgery.

   c. A male patient may experience a perceived loss of masculinity.

   d. The effect would not differ greatly between a female and a male patient.

4 In dealing with end-of-life disputes between a patient's family members, under what circumstance would it be appropriate to invoke Catholic theology?

   a. Under any circumstance; Catholics favor preservation of life.

   b. If the majority of the family is Catholic.

   c. If the patient's next of kin is Catholic.

   d. If the Catholic tradition is meaningful to the patient.

5 Which of the following words is used to describe the patient–physician relationship in the Catholic faith?

   a. "Supernatural".

   b. "Sacred".

   c. "Covenant".

   d. "Moral obligation".

6 According to the Catholic Church, what is the primary difference between "ordinary" and "extraordinary" treatment options?

   a. The amount of harm or pain caused to the patient.

   b. The amount of money spent on a given treatment.

   c. The number of steps that a treatment option takes.

   d. The degree of invasiveness of the treatment.

7 According to the Catholic Church, under what circumstance is withholding food for the comfort of the patient a morally correct action?

   a. Withholding a patient's access to nourishment is never a correct action.

   b. When giving the patient food provides a small but distinct benefit.

   c. When the patient is in excruciating pain.

   d. When nourishment no longer provides benefit for the patient.

Case 18: Juana Caban: A 21-year-old Puerto Rican woman who is pregnant and HIV-positive

Select the best answer

1 Which of the following questions is appropriate to ask a pregnant woman when taking her history?
   a. Have you and your husband started picking out baby names?
   b. Have you had any trouble looking into day care programs?
   c. Is the baby's father still part of your life?
   d. What does your husband think about your pregnancy?

2 How can a physician help ensure that a single pregnant teenager has the support she needs?
   a. Contact the patient's parents and trust them to provide support for their daughter.
   b. Ask the patient about all the important people in her day-to-day life.
   c. Help the patient track down the baby's father.
   d. Direct the patient to a social worker.

3 What is an appropriate treatment option for HIV patients in the first trimester of pregnancy?
   a. Treatment is usually delayed until the 2nd trimester.
   b. Both oral and intravenous AZT.
   c. Intravenous AZT.
   d. Oral AZT.

4 When is it acceptable for an adult patient to withhold potentially life-threatening diagnosis from his/her family?
   a. By law, the patient may make personal health decisions without telling others.
   b. It is never acceptable to withhold personal health information from family.
   c. Only if the patient is free of psychological disorders.
   d. Only if the patient's health insurance is not being paid for by his/her family.

5 According to HIPPA, to whom can physicians routinely divulge confidential patient information?
   a. Only individuals identified by the patient.
   b. Only the patient.
   c. Only the immediate family of the patient.
   d. Only one individual chosen by the patient.

6 Which of the following is an ethical obligation of physicians?
   a. Patience.
   b. Veracity.
   c. Mercy.
   d. Honor.

7 What is the ethical principle of "Beneficence" obligation?
   a. Doctor–patient discussions are privileged and confidential.
   b. Physicians should tell the truth.
   c. Physicians should act in the best interest of the patient.
   d. Patients have the right to make their own decisions.

Case 19: Alice Gregory: A 71-year-old African American woman with aortic stenosis

Select the best answer

1 Which of the following is unlikely to influence the doctor–patient relationship?
   a. The cleanliness of the office.
   b. Physician's bias toward patients.
   c. Past experiences of patients.
   d. Personal prejudices of patients against certain ethnic groups.

2 Foreign medical graduates (FMGs) constitute what percentage of physicians in the U.S.?
   a. 5%.
   b. 15%.
   c. 25%.
   d. 35%.

3 Which of the following is an accurate statement about the Educational Commission for Foreign Medical Graduates (ECFMG)?
   a. ECFMG assists with learning English as a second language.
   b. ECFMG fully prepares foreign graduates to discuss medical decision-making.
   c. Completion of the ECFMG is comparable to an immersion experience.
   d. Completion of the ECFMG may mask genuine problems with English fluency, which may affect doctor–patient communication.

4 What is the most appropriate response when a patient's behavior or comments during an office visit trigger anger or negative emotions in the physician?

   a. Confront the patient immediately.

   b. Recognize these emotions and maintain control.

   c. Ignore the comments and send in a resident to see the patient.

   d. End the visit and schedule a follow-up with another physician.

5 The ability of physicians to control their emotions and responses toward patients may positively influence which of the following?

   a. Development of rapport.

   b. Comfort level with a physical examination.

   c. Adherence to medication.

   d. Malpractice litigation.

6 Research supports that race/ethnicity concordance in the patient–physician relationship is associated with which of the following statements?

   a. Preference of patients to avoid racist physicians.

   b. Improved long-term medical outcomes.

   c. Better patient care during hospital visits.

   d. Improved partnership in decision-making and increased patient satisfaction.

7 Generally, what is the most appropriate response when a patient asks an offensive question?

   a. Remove oneself from the room to regain control of emotions.

   b. Tactfully defend one's position by involving another colleague.

   c. Initiate a respectful discussion to prevent a defensive counter-reaction.

   d. Confront the patient with a defensive response.

8 The U.S. health care system gives patients the right to choose their health care providers. How should physicians respond to requests for a provider of a certain gender, race, or ethnicity?

   a. Only take care of patients from certain ethnic groups.

   b. Refuse to accommodate these kinds of requests as they reflect a bias or prejudice.

   c. Always accommodate every patient's request.

   d. Discuss with the patient his/her reasons for this specific preference.

Case 20: Sunil Guha: A 32-year-old South Asian Indian man with metabolic syndrome

Select the best answer

1 The criteria for which of the following risk factors for metabolic syndrome varies by race/ethnicity?
   a. Hypertension.
   b. Fasting plasma glucose levels.
   c. Waist circumference.
   d. HDL-C levels.

2 Metabolic syndrome includes low HDL-C and elevated blood pressure defined in men by which of the following?
   a. HDL-C <50 mg/dL and blood pressure $\geq$120/75 mm Hg.
   b. HDL-C <40 mg/dL and blood pressure $\geq$130/85 mm Hg.
   c. HDL-C <35 mg/dL and blood pressure $\geq$135/85 mm Hg.
   d. HDL-C <30 mg/dL and blood pressure $\geq$140/90 mm Hg.

3 When assessing a patient's dietary habits, which of the following statements is the most effective approach?
   a. Assume the patient's dietary habits relate to his/her specific culture.
   b. Request that the patient record his/her food intake for 1 month.
   c. Refer the patient to a registered dietitian during the first visit.
   d. Take a detailed history of the patient's dietary preferences.

4 Which of the following is least effective in enabling patients to adhere to a healthy diet?
   a. Bringing patients back frequently for follow-up visits.
   b. Asking patients to complete food and activity records.
   c. Telling patients to eliminate certain foods without follow-up.
   d. Setting goals that target the problem areas in diet.

5 Which of the following is an important difference in the diets of Asian Indian patients in India versus Asian Indian patients living in the U.S.?
   a. Patients in the U.S. have a lower carbohydrate intake on average.
   b. Patients in the U.S. eat more curry.
   c. Patients in India use more vanaspathi (hydrogenated fat) in their cooking.
   d. Patients in India are less likely to eat pork.

6 Studies show that, in comparison to other ethnic groups in the U.S., Asian Indians are more likely to present with which of the following behaviors?
   a. Alcohol abuse.
   b. Sedentary lifestyle.
   c. Poor adherence to medication.
   d. Depression.

7 When a patient does not return for follow-up after several years, what is the most appropriate response if and when he/she does return for medical care?
   a. Confront the patient for not following up.
   b. Express disappointment to the patient for not following up.
   c. Thank the patient for returning and remain supportive.
   d. Refuse to see the patient.

8 Which of the following lifestyle changes is most likely to decrease a patient's risk of coronary heart disease?
   a. Switching from 2% milk to 1% low-fat milk.
   b. Exercising on a daily basis.
   c. Taking a multivitamin supplement.
   d. Cutting back on work schedule.

9 When advising an Asian Indian patient to reduce his/her risk for coronary heart disease, which of the following dietary changes would be the most effective?
   a. Recommend healthy substitutions for ingredients typically found in traditional food.
   b. Avoid curry, a common Indian spice.
   c. Recommend the addition of lean beef.
   d. Replace herbs in the patient's diet with salt.

Case 21: Pepper Hawthorne: A 19-year-old Caucasian woman with a stroke

Select the best answer

1 Which of the following factors is most likely to contribute to the minimization of the significance of a patient's symptoms by a health care provider?
   a. Middle age.
   b. Female gender.
   c. High income.
   d. Caucasian race.

2 "Psychologicalization of illness" is best defined by which of following statements?
   a. Redefinition of illness as an intangible process.
   b. Examination of the effects of physical illness on a patient's mental capacity.
   c. The stress response to acute illness.
   d. Overemphasis on psychological factors without just evidence.

3 Which of the following statements may be an effect of psychologicalization in the clinical context?
   a. Reduced psychological distress.
   b. Increased involvement of psychologists and psychiatrists in the management of acutely ill patients.
   c. Misdiagnosis.
   d. Increased detection of undiagnosed depression.

4 Psychologization disproportionately affects the care of patients from which of the following groups?
   a. Women.
   b. African Americans.
   c. People with low socioeconomic status.
   d. People with a history of substance abuse.

5 Which of the following approaches is most appropriate when discussing illicit drug use with patients?
   a. Asking the patient when he/she last used drugs.
   b. Ordering blood work without addressing the issue with the patient.
   c. Framing a question in a nonaccusatory and nonjudgmental manner.
   d. Discussing the issue with the patient's family instead of the patient.

6 Under what circumstances should an 18-year-old patient be excluded from the decision-making process regarding his/her health?
   a. Never; by law, patients 18 years and older make their own health care decisions.
   b. If the parents think that the patient is too immature to make appropriate decisions about his/her care.
   c. If the patient's parents choose to represent the patient.
   d. Only if the patient lacks the capacity to make medical decisions.

7 Health care decision making regarding children and adolescents under the age of 18 years should ultimately strive to develop which of the following?
   a. Ensure that the patient is informed and assents to the plan of care.
   b. Deferral of invasive procedures until the patient reaches the age of consent.
   c. Identification of an independent patient advocate outside of the family.
   d. Legal emancipation of the minor patient so he/she can make his/her own decisions.

Case 22: Alika Nkuutu: A 24-year-old African woman with sickle cell disease

Select the best answer

1 Patients from West Africa are most likely to be unfamiliar with what aspect of the U.S. health care system?
   a. Getting annual vaccinations.
   b. Scheduling follow-up appointments.
   c. Obtaining medications from a pharmacy.
   d. Having a primary care physician.

2 Patients who speak conversational English may receive the most benefit from which of the following resources?
   a. Medical information pamphlets.
   b. A skilled medical interpreter.
   c. Written prescription instructions.
   d. Free samples of prescribed medication.

3 Suspicion of which of the following behaviors may affect pain management plans, especially for patients with sickle cell disease?
   a. Spousal abuse.
   b. Heavy smoking.
   c. Recreational drug abuse.
   d. Narcotic dependence.

4 Disparities in effective pain management for racial and ethnic minorities appear most frequently under which of the following settings?
   a. Rehabilitation therapy.
   b. Physical therapy.
   c. Cancer therapy.
   d. Preoperational therapy.

5 Stereotyping of what ethnic background is significant in the discussion of sickle cell disease?

   a. African American.
   b. Asian.
   c. Hispanic (Latino).
   d. Caucasian.

6 Which of the following nonverbal cues would be deemed offensive according to West African culture?

   a. Making direct eye contact.
   b. Extending one's left hand in greeting.
   c. Shaking hands.
   d. Crossing one's legs while seated.

7 Which of the following is the best way to defuse cultural misunderstandings that serve as obstacles in cross-cultural care?

   a. Reinforce personal authority in the doctor–patient relationship.
   b. Advocate changes in current medical school curriculum.
   c. Avoid serving patients from particular backgrounds.
   d. Maintain open and honest communication with patients.

Case 23: Miguel Cortez: A 9-year-old Mexican boy with asthma

Select the best answer

1 When seeing an underage child with a parent who does not speak English, which approach would have the greatest positive impact on adherence?

   a. Using a trained medical interpreter.
   b. Providing bilingual medical pamphlets for the patient.
   c. Giving verbal instructions directly to the patient.
   d. Providing written instructions for medications.

2 Which of the following statements is true about ad hoc interpreters?

   a. They are generally preferred over using hospital employees.
   b. They almost always have experience with medical terminology.
   c. They are generally less useful than trained medical interpreters.
   d. They always contribute to better health care experiences.

3 Which of the following abilities is promoted through the use of trained medical interpreters?
   a. Ability to have "small talk" with patients.
   b. Ability to diagnose psychosocial disorders.
   c. Ability to address adherence issues.
   d. Ability to educate patients about their medications.

4 The belief that asthma treatment can lead to addiction is prevalent among which of the following groups?
   a. Chinese Americans.
   b. Dominican Americans.
   c. Mexican Americans.
   d. Columbian Americans.

5 Which of the following Hispanic groups have the highest prevalence and mortality rates of asthma compared to the others?
   a. Mexican Americans.
   b. Dominican Americans.
   c. Puerto Rican Americans.
   d. Cuban Americans.

6 Which of the following Spanish words would be most appropriate to describe "wheezing" to Mexican patients?
   a. Resuello.
   b. Sibilancia.
   c. Jadeo.
   d. Ronquer.

7 Fear of deportation among undocumented Hispanic immigrants may lead to which of the following results?
   a. Delayed medical treatment.
   b. Complete disclosure of relevant medical information.
   c. Decreased risk in asthma morbidity.
   d. Increased patient interest in personal health.

Case 24: Naomi Fulton: A 49-year-old African American woman with metabolic syndrome

Select the best answer

1 Which of the following approaches is most effective in helping patients change their diet and lifestyle?
   a. Taking a diet and exercise history.
   b. Telling patients to eat five servings of vegetables a day.
   c. Recommending daily exercise for at least 30 minutes.
   d. Emphasizing the importance of weight reduction.

2 What is the effect of weight-loss counseling by primary care providers on patient willingness to attempt to lose weight?
   a. Negligible.
   b. Doubles the odds.
   c. Triples the odds.
   d. Quadruples the odds.

3 What percentage of body weight lost represents the threshold in modifying risk factors for metabolic syndrome?
   a. 20–25%.
   b. 15–20%.
   c. 10–15%.
   d. 5–10%.

4 Which of the following approaches would be most effective in treating patients who have been unsuccessful at losing weight?
   a. Motivational interviewing.
   b. Teach back approach.
   c. Referral to a dietitian.
   d. Recommendation of self-help books.

5 Patients with low levels of conviction to change behavior should be treated using which of the following approaches?
   a. Prescribing a plan of action.
   b. Documenting the patient's current stage and waiting for a teachable moment.
   c. Attempting to persuade the patient to change his/her behavior.
   d. Reminding the patient of the long-term consequences of his/her actions.

6 It is the responsibility of the physician to reinforce which of the following concepts about medical issues and weight status?
   a. Being skinny is generally associated with better health.
   b. Body weight is ultimately a personal preference.
   c. Being overweight has many medical benefits.
   d. Excess weight around the abdomen contributes to metabolic syndrome.

7 Giving advice about diet and lifestyle change is most effective at which of the following stages?
   a. Precontemplative.
   b. Contemplative.
   c. Postcontemplative.
   d. Relapse.

8 What is the role of the health care provider in the counseling?
   a. Acts as a partner who actively listens.
   b. Helps the client explore pros and cons of change.
   c. Provides expert advice given the patient's social circumstances.
   d. Elicits motivation from the patient through conversation.

Case 25: Bobby Napier: A 68-year-old Caucasian Appalachian man with type 2 diabetes

Select the best answer

1 Which of the following choices represents a barrier to health care for low-income patients in the U.S.?
   a. Limited health care and educational programs close to home.
   b. Language proficiency.
   c. Busy schedule.
   d. Availability of brand-name medication.

2 How should physicians interact with colleagues to lower rates of poor adherance among patients?
   a. Support colleagues who have had frustrating experiences with patients.
   b. Provide feedback on communication style by reframing patient encounters.
   c. Keep tabs on patients and families who have histories of non-compliance.
   d. Reprimand colleagues for rash, unprofessional behavior.

3 Physicians should examine the ecological/environmental context of patients before which of the following?
   a. Performing a physical examination.
   b. Asking the patient to state the purpose of the visit.
   c. Meeting the patient for the first time.
   d. Discussing a therapeutic plan.

4 After taking the medical history of a patient, which of the following approaches would be most effective in eliciting the need to address personal health issues?
   a. Warn the patient of long-term consequences.
   b. Implement a plan of action immediately.
   c. Share opinions about the patient's ability to problem solve.
   d. Consult family members in the decision-making process.

5 Which of the following is common among indigent, rural Appalachian patients?

   a. Perceived socioeconomic discrimination.

   b. Lack of knowledge about preventive health care.

   c. Sexually transmitted infections.

   d. Willingness to adhere to prescribed medications.

6 When could ministers or elders from the religious community play a role in patient care?

   a. Only when the patient is put under hospice care.

   b. At the request of the patient or family member.

   c. At the request of the physician.

   d. When their involvement is welcome by the patient and their family.

7 How can physicians help patients from rural communities control their diabetes and overcome barriers in health care?

   a. By identifying diabetic outreach programs and traveling clinics.

   b. By providing medical pamphlets regarding diabetes.

   c. By referring patients to a local dietitian.

   d. By encouraging daily exercise.

8 Which of the following recommendations to combat diabetes may be unfeasible in very urban environments?

   a. Eat more fresh fruit.

   b. Do 25 jumping-jacks every morning.

   c. Go out for a walk every day.

   d. See your dietitian at least twice a year.

Answers

Case 1: The Case of Ruth Franklin

1 a
2 b
3 c
4 d
5 c
6 a
7 d
8 c

Case 2: The Case of Carl Jones

1 c
2 c
3 d
4 a
5 b
6 d
7 c
8 b

Case 3: The Case of Maria Morales

1 c
2 b
3 d

4 a
5 c
6 b
7 d
8 a

Case 4: The Case of Maya Mohammed

1 b
2 d
3 d
4 d
5 c
6 a
7 d
8 b

Case 5: The Case of Jon Le

1 b
2 c
3 d
4 b
5 c
6 d
7 a
8 b

Case 6: The Case of Nadia Rosenberg

1 b

2 a

3 b

4 d

5 c

6 a

7 b

8 b

9 a

Case 7: The Case of Isabel Delgado

1 d

2 a

3 b

4 c

5 d

6 b

7 c

8 b

Case 8: The Case of George Dennis

1 d

2 b

3 c

4 c

5 a

6 d

7 c

8 d

Case 9: The Case of Mary Jones

1 c

2 d

3 b

4 a

5 b

6 c

7 d

8 b

9 a

Case 10: The Case of Priya Krishnamurthy

1 c

2 b

3 d

4 a

5 b

6 c

7 c

8 b

9 d

Case 11: The Case of Carlos Cruz

1 a

2 b

3 d

4 c

5 b

6 d

7 c

8 a

Case 12: The Case of Denise Smith

1 a
2 c
3 d
4 b
5 a
6 c
7 d
8 b

Case 13: The Case of Mae Ling Chung

1 c
2 a
3 b
4 d
5 c
6 d
7 b
8 b

Case 14: The Case of Earl Collins

1 c
2 b
3 d
4 c
5 b
6 a
7 b

Case 15: The Case of Irma Matos

1 a
2 b
3 d
4 c
5 b
6 d
7 a
8 b

Case 16: The Case of Eileen Clark

1 a
2 c
3 a
4 c
5 c
6 d

Case 17: The Case of Leslie O'Malley

1 a
2 b
3 c
4 d
5 c
6 a
7 d

Case 18: The Case of Juana Caban

1 c
2 b
3 d
4 a
5 a
6 b
7 c

Case 19: The Case of Alice Gregory

1 a
2 c
3 d
4 b
5 a
6 d
7 c
8 d

Case 20: The Case of Sunil Guha

1 c
2 b
3 d
4 c
5 a
6 b
7 c
8 b
9 a

Case 21: The Case of Pepper Hawthorne

1 b
2 d
3 c
4 a
5 c
6 d
7 a

Case 22: The Case of Alika Nkuutu

1 c
2 b
3 d
4 c
5 a
6 b
7 d

Case 23: The Case of Miguel Cortez

1 a
2 c
3 d
4 b
5 c
6 d
7 a

Case 24: The Case of Naomi Fulton

1 a

2 c

3 d

4 a

5 b

6 d

7 b

8 a

Case 25: The Case of Bobby Napier

1 a

2 b

3 d

4 c

5 b

6 d

7 a

8 c

Index

A1. Value historical impact of racism	Domain 4: Communication Skills Specific to Cross-Culture Communication					Domain 5: Use of Interpreters			Domain 6: Self-reflection, Culture of Medicine				
A1. Value historical impact of racism	S4. Elicit information in family-centered context	S5. Use negotiating and problem-solving skills	S6. Assess and enhance adherence	A1. Respect patient's cultural beliefs	A2. Nonjudgmental listening to health beliefs	K1. Describe functions of an interpreter	K2. List effective ways of working with interpreter	S1. Identify and collaborate with an interpreter	K1. Describe the physician-patient power imbalance	S1. Recognize institutional cultural issues	S2. Engage in reflection about own beliefs	S3. Use reflective practices in patient care	A1. Value the need to address personal bias
												X	X
			X										
				X	X								
		X		X	X								
		X	X	X					X				
						X	X	X					
			X	X	X				X				
									X	X	X		
	X	X	X										
				X			X	X			X	X	
		X		X		X	X	X					
					X						X		X
	X	X											
	X	X		X	X								
X	X												
	X	X											X
	X	X											X
		X							X				
			X	X									
		X								X			
X						X							
		X				X	X	X		X			
		X											
		X		X							X	X	